Health Communication

Richard K. Thomas

Health Communication

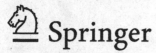 Springer

Richard K. Thomas
rthomas5@midsouth.rr.com

e-ISBN: 0-387-26116-8
e-ISBN: 978-0-387-26116-4

ISBN: 978-1-4419-3866-4

Printed on acid-free paper.

Printed in the United States of America.   (TB/SBA)

9 8 7 6 5 4 3 2 1

springeronline.com

Preface

During the last years of the 20th century health professionals developed a growing appreciation of the critical role that communication plays in healthcare. The communication of information among the various players in healthcare has always been taken as a given. Like many common phenomenon, however, the nuances and unspoken interaction may have serious implications for the communication process. Examples of the pivotal role of communication in healthcare are everywhere—communication between doctors (and other clinicians) and patients, between health educators and their clients, between pharmaceutical companies and consumers, between parents and children.

Just as important as the positive contribution that communication can make to healthcare has been the realization of the negative impact that ineffective communication can have within the healthcare arena. We only have to note the contribution of poor communication to malpractice suits, misdiagnoses, failures in patient compliance, and cross-cultural misunderstandings to see the role that communication plays.

Many of the challenges facing healthcare today, in fact, reflect failures in communication. The headlines are full of stories related to medical errors, patient confidentiality, patient compliance, and other concerns related to the delivery of care. The common theme running through these headline-grabbing issues is communication.

Given these circumstances, there has never been a better time to address the issue of health communication. It is a time when the importance of health communication is being recognized, when the role of health communication is expanding, and when the implications of effective (or ineffective) communication are becoming more significant.

There is no question that the need for stepped up efforts in the area of health communication is growing in all areas. Fortunately, the resources available for improving health communication are increasing as well. The base of knowledge—that which is being communicated—has increased exponentially over the past few years. Health professionals now know what to tell people in most instances. The body of research on what is effective and what is not has grown dramatically and health professionals are benefiting from advances in communication theory. The number and range of available communication techniques have greatly expanded, providing the health communicator with an unprecedented armamentarium of approaches to use. The dramatic impact of the Internet on our everyday lives has also ushered in an age of opportunity for those who seek to communicate health-related messages to both the general public and to narrowly targeted audiences.

The revival of interest in traditional systems of healing has also furthered the interest in health communication. The movement toward integrated health systems that take a holistic approach to the patient emphasizes the importance of communication between healers and their clients. The critical role of therapeutic communication that formed the basis for treatment within traditional systems has been rediscovered and the health communication process is increasingly being recognized as more than a technical aspect of care but as a component of the therapy process in its own right.

This renewed interest is also reflected in recent funding initiatives on the part of federal agencies. Driven by concerns over issues like access to care, disparities in treatment, and increasing patient dissatisfaction, numerous federal programs now include research on health communication among their priorities.

Ultimately, this book hopes to ride the wave of optimism with regard to the role health communication can play in improving the health status of individuals and communities. This author's presentation in the early 1980s about the imminent ascendancy of health communication in the field turned out to be premature. But today the knowledge, acceptance and tools necessary for the promotion of health communication are all in place.

University of Tennessee   Richard K. Thomas
  Health Science Center
  May 2005

Contents

Chapter 1

Introduction to Health Communication

C hapter 1 introduces the reader to the concept of health communication and defines the basic terms in the field. The sections that follow distinguish health communication from other forms of information dissemination and describe who does it and who they do it to. The organization of the book is also outlined in this chapter.

DEFINING COMMUNICATION AND HEALTH COMMUNICATION

Communication refers to the transmission or exchange of information and implies the sharing of meaning among those who are communicating. Communication serves the purposes of: 1) initiating actions, 2) making known needs and requirements, 3) exchanging information, ideas, attitudes and beliefs, 4) engendering understanding, and/or 5) establishing and maintaining relations (U.S. Office of Disease Prevention and Health Promotion, 2004). Communication, thus, plays an integral role in the delivery of healthcare and the promotion of health.

According to Healthy People 2010 guidelines, *health communication* encompasses the study and use of communication strategies to inform and influence individual and community decisions that enhance health. It links the domains of communication and health.

Health communication encompasses the study and use of communication strategies to inform and influence individual and community knowledge, attitudes and practices (KAP) with regard to health and

1

healthcare. The field represents the interface between communication and health and is increasingly recognized as a necessary element for improving both personal and public health. Health communication can contribute to all aspects of disease prevention and health promotion.

The most obvious application of health communication has been in these areas of health promotion and disease prevention. Research has uncovered improvement of interpersonal and group interactions in clinical situations (for example, between provider and patient, provider and provider, and among members of a healthcare team) through the training of health professionals and patients in effective communication skills.

Virtually all Americans have been exposed to health messages through public education campaigns that seek to change the social climate in order to encourage healthy behaviors, create awareness, change attitudes, and motivate individuals to adopt recommended behaviors. Campaigns traditionally have relied on mass communication (such as public service announcements on billboards, radio, and television) and educational messages in printed materials (such as pamphlets) to deliver health messages. Other campaigns have integrated mass media with community-based programs and/or incorporated social marketing techniques.

Increasingly, health improvement activities are taking advantage of digital technologies, such as CD-ROM and the World Wide Web, that can target audiences, tailor messages, and engage people in interactive, ongoing exchanges about health. As population-based approaches to healthcare have become more common, the role of health communication has expanded. Community-centered prevention shifts attention from the individual to group-level change and emphasizes the empowerment of individuals and communities to effect change on multiple levels.

Federal healthcare officials have emphasized the importance of health communication in addressing the nation's "leading health indicators". These focus on key health improvement activities and are described in *Healthy People 2010: Understanding and Improving Health* (2004). Movement toward the achievement of these objectives depends to a great extent on effective health communication. The promotion of regular physical activity, healthy weight, good nutrition, and responsible sexual behavior all require a range of information, education, and advocacy efforts, as does the reduction of tobacco use, substance abuse, injuries, and violence. Effective counseling and patient education geared to behavior change require healthcare providers and patients to have good communication skills. Public information campaigns are used, for example, to promote increased fruit and vegetable consumption, higher rates of preventive screening, higher rates of clinical preventive services, and increased adoption of risk-reducing behaviors.

Health communication can take place at a number of different levels, and the Centers for Disease Control and Prevention identified the following levels of impact:

The individual – The individual is the most fundamental target for health-related change, since it is individual behaviors that affect health status. Communication can affect the individual's awareness, knowledge, attitudes, self-efficacy, and skills for behavior change. Activity at all other levels ultimately aims to affect and support individual change.

The social network – An individual's relationships and the groups to which an individual belongs can have a significant impact on his or her health. Health communication programs can work to shape the information a group receives and may attempt to change communication patterns or content. Opinion leaders within a network are often a point of entry for health programs.

The organization – Organizations include formal groups with a defined structure, such as associations, clubs, and civic groups; worksites; schools; primary healthcare settings; and retailers. Organizations can carry health messages to their membership, provide support for individual efforts, and make policy changes that enable individual change.

The community – The collective well-being of communities can be fostered by creating structures and policies that support healthy lifestyles and by reducing or eliminating hazards in social and physical environments. Community-level initiatives are planned and led by organizations and institutions that can influence health: schools, worksites, healthcare settings, community groups, and government agencies.

The society – Society as a whole has many influences on individual behavior, including norms and values, attitudes and opinions, laws and policies, and the physical, economic, cultural, and information environments.

Clearly, the more levels a communication program can influence, the greater the likelihood of creating and sustaining the desired change. Health communication alone, however, cannot change systemic problems related to health, such as poverty, environmental degradation, or lack of access to health care, but comprehensive health communication programs should include a systematic exploration of all the factors that contribute to health and the strategies that could be used to influence these factors. Well-designed health communication activities can help individuals better understand their own and their communities' needs so that they can take appropriate actions to maximize health.

THE ROLE OF COMMUNICATION

One of the major developments of recent years has been the "discovery" of the role that health communication can play (for good and bad) in determining individual and community health status. Effective communication can (a) improve the health outcomes of acute and chronic conditions, (b) reduce the impact of racial, ethnic, disease-specific and socioeconomic factors in care, and (c) improve the effectiveness of prevention and health promotion. The large gap between expected and achieved quality in health care can be attributed to ineffective communication between providers and patients and their families, providers and providers, health care organizations and providers (Institute of Medicine, 2001). Similarly, the large gaps in quality between whites and minorities that are not explainable by differences in insurance or socioeconomic status reflect the crucial role that inadequate communication and lack of cultural competence play.

Health communication has become an accepted tool for promoting public health. Health communication principles are often used today for various disease prevention and control strategies including advocacy for health issues, marketing health plans and products, educating patients about medical care or treatment choices, and educating consumers about healthcare quality issues. At the same time, the availability of new technologies and computer-based media is expanding access to health information and raising questions about equality of access, accuracy of information, and effective use of these new tools.

The many roles that health communication can play have been highlighted by the Centers for Disease Control and Prevention. These roles include:

- Increase knowledge and awareness of a health issue, problem, or solution
- Influence perceptions, beliefs, attitudes, and social norms
- Prompt action
- Demonstrate or illustrate skills
- Show the benefit of behavior change
- Increase demand for health services
- Reinforce knowledge, attitudes, and behavior
- Refute myths and misconceptions
- Help coalesce organizational relationships
- Advocate for a health issue or a population group

Many patients report that they are not satisfied with the quality of their interactions with healthcare professionals. Significant gaps in communication between patients and healthcare professionals are evident in the general population. These gaps are more pronounced among (a) marginalized groups such as those with disabilities, low literacy, limited English proficiency or low socioeconomic status, (b) stigmatized groups such as those with HIV infection, obesity, or mental illnesses, and (c) minority populations such as African-Americans and refugees (University of Rochester Medical Center, 2004).

Poor communication has a strongly negative impact on outcomes of (a) chronic diseases including diabetes and hypertension, (b) acute illnesses, including pain control, morbidity following surgery, and length of hospital stay, and (c) mental illnesses such as depression and schizophrenia.

Improvements in communication in healthcare settings, invariably lead to better health outcomes. Furthermore, these changes may contribute to greater equity in health and healthcare for racial, ethnic, socioeconomic, educational and minority populations. Better communication can lead to improvements in prevention, motivation for behavior change, and adherence to treatment.

OBJECTIVES OF THE BOOK

One book obviously cannot transmit everything that is important about health communication and this one does not attempt that. This book is intended as an introduction to the field offering, on the one hand, an overview of this emerging discipline and, on the other, enough nuts-and-bolts information to allow the reader to further explore the field from a position of knowledge. The reader is exposed to the "why", "what", "where" and "when" of health communication, as well as the "who" and the "how". The how-to sections provide guidelines for developing health communication initiatives, and the case studies provide concrete examples. Ultimately, it is hoped that the book provides the wherewithal for transferring the growing body of knowledge on health behavior to the arena of the practitioner.

The audience for the proposed book includes a number of different constituents. A growing number of health professionals are focusing on health communication as a specialty, in addition to the significant number of individuals involved in healthcare marketing in some form or another. Students in the fields of communication, public health, healthcare administration and marketing should find this book useful, along with practitioners and consultants in those fields. Health professionals in both the public and private sectors involved in program planning, administration or evaluation should also benefit from this book.

This book focuses on the concepts, theories, and applications of health communication in the contemporary healthcare environment. The book is designed to fill a void in the literature on this topic by providing a comprehensive yet in-depth treatment of the emerging field of health communication. It is geared to the needs of both the academic and professional communities and addresses the disconnect between existing research and its application to the healthcare system.

The book could be useful as both a reference work and as a classroom text. It describes a practical approach for planning and implementing health communication efforts; it offers guidelines, not hard and fast rules. Virtually everyone in healthcare must be familiar with these concepts in today's environment, regardless of the aspect of healthcare with which they deal.

APPROACH OF THE BOOK

The approach taken by this book carries the reader through an introduction to health communication, defining the issues and reviewing the evolution of the concept. This is followed in Chapter 2 which discusses social and cultural considerations with implications for health communication, while Chapter 3 deals with the changing healthcare context. Chapter 4 covers the history of the field of health communication, linking it to the evolving healthcare arena. Chapter 5 focuses on the various audiences for healthcare, addressing the identification and profiling of target populations. These chapters are followed by Chapter 6 on the theoretical framework for communication and Chapter 7 on theories of health behavior.

With this foundation laid, Chapter 8 outlines a process for developing health communication initiatives, including goals of health communication, necessary ingredients, and critical steps in the process. The two chapters that follow describe techniques for health communication—Chapter 9 on traditional techniques for health communication and Chapter 10 on contemporary approaches to communicating health information. Chapter 11 describes procedures to be utilized in evaluating the success of communication efforts. This is followed in Chapter 12 by a number of case studies illustrating various aspects of health communication. The book ends with a discussion of the future of health communication and the factors that will influence the course of the field in the 21st century in Chapter 13.

The book contains numerous sidebars focusing on aspects of the topic that require special attention. Case examples throughout supplement the chapter devoted to case studies. Lists of additional resources (including Internet links) supplement the bibliographical listings and the glossary represents a useful resource.

References

The Institute of Medicine. (2001). *Crossing the quality chasm: A new health system for the 21st century*. Washington: National Academies Press.

US Office of Disease Prevention and Health Promotion. (2004). "Health Communication", *Healthy People 2010* (vol. 1). URL: http://healthy-people.gov/Document/HTML/volume1/11 HealthCom.htm#_edn4. Accessed on 9/20/04.

University of Rochester. (2004). URL: http://urmc.rochester.edu/fammed/comm.htm. Accessed on 1/5/05.

US Office of Disease Prevention and Promotion. (2004). Health communication, *Healthy People 2010* (vol. 1). URL: http://healthy people.gov/Document/HTML/volume1/11 HealthCom.htm#_edn4. Accessed on 9/20/04.

Additional Resources

Kreps, Gary L., & Barbara C. Thornton. (1992). *Health communication: Theory and practice* (2nd ed.). Long Grove, IL: Waveland Press.

Rice, R. E., & Atkin, C. K. (2000). *Public communication campaigns* (3rd ed.). Thousand Oaks, CA: Sage.

Thornton, Barbara C., and Gary L. Kreps. (1992). *Perspectives on health communication*. Long Grove, IL: Waveland Press.

Internet Resources

http://sla.purdue.edu/healthcomm/Introduction.html

Chapter 2

The Changing Sociocultural Context

C hapter 2 emphasizes the importance of the sociocultural context for effectively communicating health information. An understanding of the social and cultural framework of U.S. society is essential given the implications of cultural conceptions and perceptions for health communication. Current societal trends that are expected to impact the health communication process and the implications of sociocultural factors for health communication are discussed in this chapter.

THE SOCIOCULTURAL CONTEXT

Several developments in U.S. society and in healthcare over the last quarter century have laid the foundation for an expanded role for health communication, and current trends in healthcare are magnifying the importance of this role. Changes in demographic characteristics, lifestyles and other population attributes are all contributing to the growing significance of health communication.

In order to effectively transmit health information, health professionals must understand the healthcare system, and the healthcare system of any society can only be understood within the sociocultural context of that society. No two healthcare delivery systems are exactly alike, with the differences primarily a function of the contexts within which they exist. The social structure of a society, along with its cultural values, establishes the parameters for the healthcare system. In this sense, the form and function of a healthcare system reflect the form and function of the society in which it resides. Ultimately, the attributes of communication in healthcare reflect the characteristics of both that institution and the society in which it exists.

Like other institutions, healthcare establishes rules that guide the behavior of individuals within the institutional context. For example, there are guidelines for living a long, healthy life. If citizens don't follow these rules, they risk sickness and death. These guidelines are often codified in the form of "doctor's orders." Since individuals in a free society cannot be forced to live a healthy lifestyle, the healthcare institution invokes various legal and regulatory contrivances to enforce its requirements. Thus, all individuals are required to obtain certain childhood immunizations, addicts may be forced to enter rehabilitation, and patients with contagious diseases are isolated from the rest of society.

On another level, there are "rules" stating that health plan enrollees must have insurance before being treated by certain healthcare providers, that patients must receive annual checkups in order to maintain their low insurance premiums, and that individuals involved in risky activities must pay higher premiums for insurance. While there is no formal "plan" for encouraging or discouraging the behaviors that support the healthcare system, various parties, appearing to act in their own self-interest, contribute to the goals of the healthcare institution through the promulgation of such rules.

While social institutions achieve a certain permanence in a society, they must also maintain the flexibility to adjust to changing conditions. Healthcare is an excellent example of this situation. As will be seen later, no other institution has experienced the dramatic changes that healthcare experienced during the twentieth century. At the start of that century, healthcare was a very rudimentary institution with limited visibility and little credibility in society. Hospitals were considered to be places where people went to die, and doctors were to be avoided at all costs. Indeed, there was little the doctor could do for the patient anyway, and few patients were willing to take a doctor "at his word". There was no agreement on the nature of health and illness, and scientists were only beginning to understand the nature of disease. Healthcare was not even on the national radar screen for the first half of the twentieth century and accounted for a negligible amount of the gross national product.

Contrast that to the healthcare institution at the end of the twentieth century. Not only has the institution become well established in the United States, but it has come to play a dominant role in American society. The importance of the institution had become such that sociologists often referred to the "medicalization" of American society. Indeed, there are few members of contemporary U.S. society that are not under some type of medical management. In the last half of the twentieth century, the healthcare institution came to be accorded high prestige and to exert a major influence over other institutions. At the beginning of the twenty-first century health-care can claim 15 percent of the gross national product and 10 percent of the nation's workforce.

The ascendancy of the healthcare institution in the twentieth century was given impetus by a growing dependence by Americans on formal organizations of all types. The industrialization and urbanization occurring in the United States reflected a transformation from a traditional, agrarian society to a complex, modern society in which change, not tradition, was the central theme. In such a society, formal solutions to societal needs take precedence over informal responses.

The size of the healthcare institution has attracted substantial re-sources from other industrial sectors, and healthcare is an unavoidable issue in political contests. Indeed, the pharmaceutical industry, insurance industry, the American Medical Association, and the American Hospi-tal Association are among the major political lobbying groups. Further, much of our educational system is devoted to the training of health per-sonnel. The fact that the federal government has become responsible for the majority of personal healthcare expenditures illustrates the influence of healthcare on the central government.

Perhaps more telling has been the extent to which the healthcare insti-tution has been successful in the medicalization of everyday life. During the "golden age" of medicine in the 1960s and 1970s, the success of medicine resulted in an expansion of the scope of the field and led it to encom-pass various conditions that heretofore had not been considered medical matters. Thus, "conditions" like drug and alcohol abuse, homosexuality, hyperactivity in children, and obesity came to be defined as medical prob-lems. This served to increase the breadth of influence of the healthcare in-stitution, increase the prestige accorded to its representatives, and garner grant funds and other sources of wealth for the institution's representa-tives. (Expansion of this magnitude, one would imagine, would require an exponential increase in the amount of communication related to health issues. On the contrary, the success of organized medicine in gaining dom-inance over the field led in some ways to a reduction in the amount of open communication.)

Just as Americans had turned to formal educational, political and eco-nomic systems for meeting their social needs, they began to turn to a for-mal healthcare system to meet their health needs. The transformation of American society in the twentieth century clearly affected the provision of healthcare, as the traditional managers of sickness and death–the fam-ily and the church–gave way to more formal responses to health prob-lems. The health of the population became in part the responsibility of the economic, educational, and political systems and, eventually, of a fully

developed and powerful healthcare system. Traditional, informal responses to health problems gave way to complex, institutional responses.
"High touch" home remedies could not compete in an environment that
valued high-tech (and subsequently high status) responses to health problems.

Americans increasingly turned to the healthcare institution in the late
twentieth century as the solution for a wide range of social, psychological
and even spiritual issues, and physicians came to be regarded as experts
in regard to virtually any human problem. This expansion of scope is evidenced by the fact that less than half of the people in a general practitioner's
waiting room suffer from a clear-cut medical problem. They are there because of emotional disorders, sexual dysfunction, social adjustment issues,
nutritional problems, or some other non-clinical threat to their well-being.
Despite the fact that physicians are generally not trained to deal with these
conditions, the healthcare system is seen as an appropriate place to seek
solutions to these and many other non-medical maladies.

A fourth measure of the importance of an institution in an age of
media overkill is the amount of "air time" allocated to various aspects of
the society. Certainly, Americans continue to be deluged by advertisements
for all manner of consumer goods, and many of these goods take the form
of healthcare products. The most obvious change over the past decade or
two is the explosion of advertisements and paid programming related
to health, beauty and fitness. A tally of television advertisements would
indicate the extent to which health products and services have come to
dominate advertising venues. Paid programming featuring fitness training
and cable television channels devoted solely to health issues indicate the
extent to which the healthcare institution has gained ascendancy. Thus,
healthcare marketing in the mass media has grown from a cottage industry
in the postwar years to a major player in electronic media.

The increase in the visibility of health communication has been accompanied by an explosion of health information on the Internet. There
are purportedly more sites devoted to healthcare than there are to any
other topic. Increasing numbers of healthcare consumers are turning to
the World Wide Web for their healthcare information, and the health content of the Internet is playing a growing role in consumer decision-making.
The consumer interest in cyber-information has been accompanied by an
explosion in Internet-based marketing on the part of healthcare organizations. Once considered primarily a vehicle for providing information on
the part of hospitals, health plans, pharmaceutical companies, and consumer products companies, the Internet has now become a major medium
for health communication of all types.

All things considered, healthcare was the up-and-coming institution
of the second half of the twentieth century. The growing significance of

health for our personal lives and healthcare's growing role in the public arena cannot be denied. Indeed, many corporations have indicated that health benefits are one of their single largest costs. The increasing involvement of U.S. citizens in the use of health services and our annual per capita expenditures on healthcare set the U.S. apart from other countries and substantially contribute to the need for effective health communication.

THE CULTURAL "REVOLUTION" AND HEALTHCARE

The restructuring of U.S. institutions during the 20th century was accompanied by a cultural "revolution" resulting in extensive value reorientation within American society. The values associated with traditional societies that emphasized kinship, community, authority, and primary relationships became overshadowed by the values of modern industrialized societies, such as secularism, urbanism, and self-actualization. Ultimately, the restructuring of American values was instrumental in the emergence of healthcare as an important institution. These value shifts had significant implications for methods of communication as well.

The "modern" values that emerged within the U.S. after World War II supported the development of a healthcare system that would spawn modern "Western" medicine. These values shifted the emphasis in American society to economic success, educational achievement, and scientific and technological advancement. These values also supported the ascendancy of healthcare as a dominant institution during the last half of that century.

Other values became important as American culture evolved in the twentieth century. For example, change became recognized as a value in its own right. Americans came to value change and frequently sought changes in residences, jobs, partners and lifestyles. At the same time an activist orientation emerged that called for individuals to take a proactive approach to all issues, including healthcare. The aggressive approach taken by Americans in the face of health problems reflects this activist orientation.

The conceptualization of "health" as a distinct value in U.S. society represented a major development in the emergence of the healthcare institution. Prior to World War II health was generally not recognized as a value by Americans but was vaguely tied in with other notions of well-being. Public opinion polls prior to the war did not identify personal health as an issue for the U.S. populace, nor was healthcare delivery considered a societal concern. By the 1960s, however, personal health had climbed to the top of the public opinion polls as a concern, and the adequate provision of health services became an important issue in the mind of the American public. By the last third of the twentieth century, Americans had become obsessed with health as a value and with the importance of institutional solutions to health problems.

Once health became established as a value, it was a short step to establishing a formal healthcare system as the institutional means for achieving that value. An environment was created that encouraged the emergence of a powerful institution that supported many other contemporary American values. Some of them, like the value placed on human life, were considered immutable. The ethos promoted by the emerging scientific, technological and research communities contributed to the growth of the industry. The value that Americans came to place on youth, beauty and self-actualization further contributed to an expansion of the role of healthcare. The ability of the nascent healthcare system to capitalize on emerging U.S. values and garner support from the economic, political, and educational institutions assured the ascendancy of this new institutional form.

One of the major implications of shifting American values has been changing consumer attitudes. Although patterns of consumer attitudes in U.S. society tend to be complex, it is clear that a new orientation toward healthcare emerged during the second half of the twentieth century. The "patient" became transformed into a "consumer", creating a new entity with the combined expectations of a traditional patient and a contemporary customer. This consumer was much more knowledgeable about the healthcare system, much more open to innovative approaches, and much more intent on playing an active role in the diagnostic, therapeutic and health maintenance processes than any previous generation.

These new attitudes were most clearly associated with the under-50 population and certain demographically distinct groups. The movement toward gaining control of one's health was spearheaded by the baby boom cohort that is now beginning to face the chronic conditions associated with "middle age". This is the population that has been responsible for the success of health maintenance organizations, urgent care centers and birthing centers. This is the group that has been influential in limiting the discretion and control of physicians and hospitals. This cohort has also provided the impetus for the rise of "alternative therapy" as a competitor for mainstream allopathic medicine.

The approach to healthcare favored by the baby boom population is more patient centered than the traditional approach and is more likely to emphasize non-medical aspects of healthcare. In general, baby boomers are less trusting of professionals and institutions and are control oriented to the point of stubbornness. This group is more self-reliant when it comes to healthcare than previous generations and places greater value on self care and home care. It is both outcomes oriented and cost sensitive. It is a generation that prides itself in getting results and extracting value for its expenditures. While this cohort began influencing the healthcare system by "voting with its feet" during the 1980s, its members are increasingly in the positions of power that allow them to influence the reshaping of the healthcare landscape.

Perhaps more than any other trait, this population cohort is information hungry. They grew up in the "information age" and many of them entered occupations that involved knowledge management. This cohort prides itself on its communication skills and believes that knowledge is power. It is this hunger for information that makes baby boomers "good" patients in some respects and "bad" patients in others. No other cohort has been as aggressive in seeking out information as the boomers.

To a certain extent, these new attitudes toward healthcare reflect the rise of consumerism affecting all segments of society. Increasingly seeing themselves as customers rather than patients, Americans expect to receive adequate information, demand to participate in healthcare decisions that directly affect them, and insist that the healthcare they receive to be of the highest possible quality. Consumers want to receive their healthcare close to their homes, with minimal interruption to their family life and work schedules. They also want to maximize the value that they receive for their healthcare expenditures. The transformation of baby boomers from "patients" to "consumers" clearly has significant implications for health communication.

DEMOGRAPHIC TRENDS AND THEIR IMPLICATIONS FOR HEALTH COMMUNICATION

The U.S. population experienced a number of dramatic demographic trends during the last half of the twentieth century. These demographic trends are important in that they have contributed to the changing composition of the U.S. population; this, in turn, has influenced the morbidity profile of that population. Indeed, the demographic transformation of the American population in the twentieth century might be considered a major, if not the major, determinant of the needs to be addressed by the healthcare system. The impact of these trends extended beyond changes in age structure and racial composition and resulted in radically changed attitudes on the part of healthcare consumers.

These demographic trends also triggered the "epidemiologic transition" that took place in the U.S. in the second half of the twentieth century. Throughout recorded history, acute health conditions had constituted the major health threat and the leading causes of death for any population. Communicable, infectious and parasitic conditions, accidents, complications of childbirth and other acute conditions were a constant companion to human beings. At the beginning of the last century, the leading causes of death were tuberculosis, influenza, and other communicable diseases. As the mortality rate for the American population declined during the twentieth century and life expectancy increased, a significant change occurred in the morbidity and mortality profile of the population (Omran, 1971).

During the second half of the twentieth century, the changing demographic profile engendered a shift away from acute conditions and toward chronic conditions as the predominant form of health problem. Improved living conditions, better nutrition and higher standards of living, accompanied by advances in medical science, reduced or eliminated the burden of disease from acute conditions. This void was filled, however, by the emergence of chronic conditions as the leading health problems and leading causes of death. The older population that resulted from these developments was now plagued by hypertension, arthritis, and diabetes, as well as numerous conditions that reflected the lifestyles characterizing the American population in the second half of that century.

This section cannot begin to address all of the demographic trends that have contributed to the changing healthcare environment. It focuses on the key demographic trends and notes their likely implications for health communication.

Changing Age Structure

The first, and perhaps most important, demographic trend in the U.S. is the population's changing age structure. The aging of America has obviously been one of the most publicized demographic trends in history. The implications of this trend for health services demand have been well documented, with age arguably the single most important predictor of the use of health services.

The restructuring of the age distribution of the population has particular significance for the demand for health services. Population growth within the older age cohorts (age 55 and above), and particularly among the oldest-old (age 85 and over), is currently faster than that for the younger cohorts. The total U.S. population increased by 13.2 percent between 1990 and 2000, while the population 85 and over increased by over 36 percent. The movement of the baby boomers into the "middle ages" will make the largest age cohort the 45–65 age group in the first decade of the twenty-first century. Some younger cohorts (i.e., those 25–34) actually experienced a net loss of population during the 1990s. A continued "shortage" of younger working age individuals (i.e., those 25–40) will persist throughout the first decade of the 21st century, until the baby boom echo cohort enters this age group around 2010 (U.S. Census Bureau, 2003).

The factor above with the most significant implications for future healthcare demand is the movement of the huge baby boom cohort into the middle age. The first of some 77 million baby boomers are now turning 60. This is a cohort that grew up in affluence and comfort and they are used to having things, including their health, in working order. When they have to contend with the onset of chronic disease and the natural deterioration that comes with aging, the healthcare system will be significantly impacted. This is a cohort that grew up during the "marketing era" and is more comfortable with healthcare marketing than any previous generation. As will been seen later, this is also a very "savvy" consumer population that requires special consideration when it comes to health communication.

The nature of the future senior population will be determined to a great extent by the characteristics of the baby boomers. Boomers are determined to reinvent retirement, a process that appears to already be underway. Retirement is no longer seen as a type of "default" condition, but as a context for new and different lifestyles. Boomers, in fact, have already influenced the healthcare delivery system in significant ways, and now they are driving the demand for a wide range of new services such as laser eye surgery, skin rejuvenation, and menopause management.

An automatic accompaniment to the aging of America has been the feminization of its population. The changing age distribution has important implications for the population's male/female ratio. Generally speaking, the older the population, the greater the "excess" of females. Except for the very youngest ages, females outnumber males in every age cohort. Among seniors, females outnumber males two to one, and, at the oldest ages, there may be four times as many women as men. This results in an older age structure for women, and in 2000 the median age for women was 38.0 years compared to 36.5 years for men. Further, 23.2 percent of the female population was 55 or over, compared to 18.9 percent of the male population. In 2000, the excess of females over males in the population amounted to over five million in the United States.

These statistics on the female population have important implications for health communication. The female healthcare "market" is considerably larger than the male market. Further, women are more aggressive users of health services than are men. Perhaps even more important, women bear much of the burden for healthcare decision making, not only for themselves but for their families. They are also more likely to influence the health behavior of their peers. Thus, a growing body of health communication "lore" highlights women as both healthcare consumers and healthcare decision makers.

Growing Racial and Ethnic Diversity

Another demographic trend that characterized American society during the last half of the twentieth century was increasing racial and ethnic diversity. America has once again become a nation of immigrants, with the numbers of newcomers from foreign lands during the 1990s equaling historic highs. In addition, long-established ethnic and racial minorities are growing at faster rates than are native-born whites. The cumulative effect of the trends of the past several years has been a diminishing of the relative size of the white population (especially the non-Hispanic white population) and the growing significance of the black, Asian and Hispanic components of the U.S. population. The 2000 census revealed an America that was becoming less "white", with increases noted in the African-American, Asian-American/Pacific Islander, and American Indian/Alaskan Native populations as a percent of the total. More importantly, the census documented the rapid growth of the Hispanic population and by 2001 Hispanics had surpassed African Americans as a percentage of the U.S. population. Since most of the population growth during the next two decades will be a function of immigration, the proportion of non-Hispanic whites within the population will continue to decline.

Given the fact that the U.S. healthcare system has historically been geared to the needs of the mainstream white population, the trend toward greater racial and ethnic diversity can not help but have major implications for the nature of the system. Any health communication effort must take into consideration the changing racial and ethnic characteristics of the population and the demands that these changes will make on the system. This issue is made all the more important by the documented level of disparities among racial and ethnic groups in the U.S. Many factors contribute to the high rate of disparities among these groups in terms of health status, health behavior, and type of treatment by health professionals. Communication (or the lack thereof) plays no small part in the perpetuation of these inequities.

Changing Household and Family Structure

Another demographic development characterizing U.S. society is its changing household and family structure. For decades, the American family has been undergoing change. First it was high divorce rates, then it was less people marrying (and those who did marry marrying at a later age); then it was less people having children (and those that did having children had fewer of them and at a later age).

In 2000, the census reported that 54.4 percent of the U.S. population over 15 was married, a very low figure by historical standards. Some 27.1 percent had never married, 11.9 percent were separated or divorced, and 6.6 percent were widowed. These figures for the non-married categories all represent record highs. Given that health status and health behavior differs considerably among the various marital statuses, the current

and future array of statuses should be a concern for the health communicator (U.S. Census Bureau, 2003).

These changes in marital status have had major implications for the
U.S. household structure. It has meant that what is popularly considered
the "typical" American family (with two parents and x number of children)
has become a rarity, accounting for only 24 percent of the households in
2000. Today, married couple (without children) households have become
the most common household form, but this type of household accounts
for less than 28 percent of the total. "Non-traditional" households are becoming the norm, and an unprecedented proportion of households are
one-person households.

As with marital status, the changing household structure has important implications for both health status and health behavior. The demands
placed on the healthcare system by two-parent families, single-parent families, and elderly people living alone are significantly different from each
other and require different responses on the part of the healthcare system
(and, by extension, in the approach to health communication). To a great
extent, health services have been historically geared to the needs of "traditional" households involving two parents and one or more children. This
has been encouraged by the availability of employer-sponsored insurance
that focused on the wage-earning head of household. The continued di-
versification of U.S. household types for the foreseeable future is likely to
require commensurate modifications in the healthcare delivery system.

The role of the family in health communication has long been recognized. Most Americans indicate that they obtain the majority of their
information related to healthcare from informal networks of family and
friends. As these channels for health communication have become less
available due to the changing family structure, new sources for communicating health information must be established.

The direction that health communication takes in the future will be to
a great extent a reflection of the trends that characterize American society
and healthcare. The social practices, values, attitudes and lifestyles characterizing members of society will dictate the channels, messages and strategies that are utilized by health communicators.

References

Omran, A. R. (1971). The epidemiologic transition: A theory of the epidemiology of
      population change," *Milbank Memorial Quarterly*, 49, 515ff.
Thomas, Richard K. (2004). *Marketing health services*. Chicago: Health Administration Press.
US Census Bureau, US Department of Commerce, Washington, DC. "American Factfinder"
      at URL: http://census.gov. Accessed on 4/15/03.

Chapter 3

The Changing Healthcare Context

C hapter 3 highlights the role that the healthcare context plays in determining the form that communication takes. In order to set the stage, an overview of the U.S. healthcare system is provided, and the changing nature of both the healthcare system and the healthcare consumer is described. Current trends in healthcare that are expected to impact the health communication process are discussed.

U.S. HEALTHCARE IN HISTORICAL PERSPECTIVE

It is not appropriate to speak of a modern healthcare system in the United States until after World War II. Prior to that time, healthcare as an institution was poorly developed and accounted for a negligible proportion of societal resources. It remained an institutional non-entity until the period following the war when it began a rapid rise to become a major U.S. institution. Consequently, any serious consideration of health communication would date from that point as well.

The development of the healthcare system following World War II can be divided into five stages, roughly equating to the five decades of the last half of the twentieth century. As will be seen, the approach to health communication reflects the stage at which healthcare existed at a particular point in time. Each of these stages will be briefly discussed in turn.

The 1950s: The Emergence of "Modern" Medicine. As American society entered a new period of growth and prosperity following the end of World War II, the modern U.S. healthcare system began to take shape. The economic growth of the period resulted in demand for a wide range of goods and services, including healthcare. "Health" was coming to be recognized as a value in its own right, and considerable resources were expended on a fledging healthcare system that had lain dormant during the war.

The 1950s witnessed the first significant involvement of the federal government in healthcare, as the Hill-Burton Act resulted in the construction of hundreds of hospitals to meet pent up demand. Health insurance was becoming common and, spurred by the influence of trade unions, healthcare benefits became a major issue at the bargaining table.

World War II had also served as a giant "laboratory" for pioneering a wide range of medical and surgical procedures. Trauma surgery was essentially unknown prior to the war, and trauma and burn treatment capabilities were now available to apply in a civilian context. New drug therapies were being introduced and formal health services were coming to be seen as a solution for an increasing number of problems.

The 1960s: The Golden Age of American Medicine. During the 1960s the healthcare institution in the U.S. experienced unprecedented expansion in personnel and facilities. The hospital emerged as the center of the system, and the physician–much maligned in earlier decades–came to occupy the pivotal role in the treatment of disease. Physician salaries and the prestige associated with their positions grew astronomically.

Private insurance became widespread, offered primarily through employer-sponsored plans. The Medicare and Medicaid programs were introduced, and these initiatives expanded access to healthcare (at government expense) to the elderly and poor, respectively.

New therapeutic techniques were being developed, accompanied by growth in the variety of technologies and support personnel required. New conditions (e.g., alcoholism, hyperactivity) were identified as appropriate for medical treatment, resulting in an increasing proportion of the population coming under "medical management". Complete consumer trust existed in the healthcare system in general and in hospitals and physicians in particular.

The only dissension was heard on the part of those few who had discovered that certain segments of the population were not sharing in this "golden age". Even here, though, there was virtually no criticism of the disease theory system that underlay the delivery system. It was felt that the infrastructure was sound and that only some improvement in execution by the system was required to address the deficiencies.

The 1970s: Questioning the System. Entering the 1970s the healthcare system maintained a trajectory of expansion and growth. New medical procedures continued to be introduced, and there appeared to be no limit to the application of technology. Even more new conditions were identified, and increasing numbers of citizens were brought under medical management financed through private insurance and government-subsidized insurance plans. The hospital was entrenched as the focal point of the system, and the physician continued to control more than 80% of expenditures for health services.

During the 1970s, however, a number of issues began to be raised concerning the healthcare system and its operation. Issues of access and equity that were first voiced in the 1960s reached a point where they could no longer be ignored. Large segments of the population appeared to be excluded from mainstream medicine. Further, the effectiveness of the system in dealing with the overall health status of the population was brought into question. Health status indicators showed that the U.S. population was lagging behind other comparable countries in improving its health status.

The critical issue that developed in the 1970s centered on the cost of care. Clearly, the U.S. had the world's most expensive healthcare system. The costs were high and they were increasing much faster than those in other sectors of the economy. While it was once assumed that resources for the provision of healthcare were infinite, it came to be realized that there was a limit on what could be spent to provide health services. Coupled with questions about access and effectiveness, the escalating cost of care was a basis for widespread alarm.

During this period the underlying foundation of the healthcare system was questioned for the first time. Earlier criticism had been directed at the operation of the system, and it was assumed that the disease theory system was appropriate. Hence, a "band-aid" approach had been advocated rather than major surgery. As the 1970s ended, more and more voices were being raised concerning the basic assumptions underlying the system.

The 1980s: The Great Transformation.   The 1980s will no doubt be seen by historians as a watershed for U.S. healthcare. The numerous issues that had been emerging over the previous two decades came to a head as the 1980s began. By the end of the decade, American healthcare had become almost unrecognizable to veteran health professionals. Virtually every aspect of the system had undergone transformation and a new paradigm began to emerge as the basis for the disease theory system.

The escalating–and seemingly uncontrollable–costs associated with healthcare care prompted the Medicare administration to introduce the prospective payment system. Other insurers soon followed suit with a variety of cost containment methods. Employers, who were footing much of the bill for increasing healthcare costs, began to take a more active role in the management of their plans.

The decade also witnessed the introduction of new financial arrangements and organizational structures. Experiments abounded in an attempt to find ways to more effectively and efficiently provide health services. The major consequence of these activities was the introduction of managed care as an approach to controlling the utilization of services and, ultimately, the cost borne by insurers. The managed care concept called for incentives on the part of all parties for more appropriate use of the system.

This development resulted in considerable shifts in both power and risk within the system. The power that resided in hospital administrators and physicians was blamed for much of the cost and inefficiency that existed. Third-party payors, employers and consumers began to attempt to share in this power. Large groups of purchasers emerged that began to negotiate for lower costs in exchange for their "wholesale" business. Insurers, who had historically borne most of the financial risk involved in the financing of health services, began shifting some of this risk to providers and consumers.

Developments outside of healthcare were also having significant influence. Chief among these was the changing nature of the American population. The acute conditions that had dominated the healthcare scene since the inception of modern medicine were being supplanted by the chronic conditions characteristic of an older population. The respiratory conditions, parasitic diseases and playground injuries of earlier decades were being replaced in the physician's waiting room by arthritis, hypertension and diabetes. The mismatch between the capabilities of the healthcare system and the needs of the patients it was designed to serve became so severe that a new disease theory system began to emerge.

The 1990s: The Shifting Paradigm. Although change occurs unevenly throughout a system as complex as American healthcare, many are arguing that by the late 1990s a true paradigm shift was occurring. Simply put, this involved a shift from an emphasis on "medical care" to one on "healthcare". *Medical care* is narrowly defined in terms of the formal services provided by the healthcare system and refers primarily to those functions of the healthcare system that are under the influence of medical doctors. This concept focuses on the clinical or treatment aspects of care, and excludes the non-medical aspects of healthcare. *Healthcare* refers to any function that might be directly or indirectly related to preserving, maintaining, and/or enhancing health status. This concept includes not only formal activities (such as visiting a health professional) but also such informal activities as preventive care (e.g., brushing teeth), exercise, proper diet, and other health maintenance activities.

Since the 1970s there has been a steady movement of activities and emphasis away from medical care toward healthcare. The importance of the non-medical aspects of care has become increasingly appreciated. The growing awareness of the connection between health status and lifestyle and the realization that medical care is limited in its ability to control the disorders of modern society have prompted a move away from a strictly medical model of health and illness to one that incorporates more of a social and psychological perspective (Engle 1977).

Despite this changing orientation, an imbalance remains in the system with regard to the allocation of resources to its various components. Treatment still commands the lion's share of the healthcare dollar, and most research is still focused on developing cures rather than preventive measures. The hospital remains the focal point of the system, and the physician continues to be its primary gatekeeper. Nevertheless, each of these underpinnings of medical care was substantially weakened during the 1980s, with a definitive shift toward a healthcare-oriented paradigm evident during the 1990s.

At the close of the twentieth century, the healthcare institution continued to be beset by many problems. It could be argued that the system was too expensive, particularly in view of its inability to effectively address contemporary health problems and raise the overall health status of the population, and that large segments of the population were excluded from mainstream medicine. The fact that "administrative costs" account for some 30 percent of the U.S. healthcare dollar (compared to less than 10 percent in socialized systems) suggested that there were considerable inefficiencies in the system.

2000–2010: New Millennium Healthcare.   As the twenty-first century dawns, U.S. healthcare appears to be entering yet another phase, one that reflects both late twentieth century developments and newly emerging trends. The further entrenchment of the "healthcare" paradigm appears to be occurring, as the medical model continues to lose its salience. This trend is driven in part by the resurgence of consumerism that is being witnessed and the reemergence of a consumer-choice market. At the same time, financial exigencies and consumer demand are encouraging more holistic, less intensive approaches to care.

The new millennium is witnessing continued disparities in healthcare, exacerbated by the growing number of uninsured individuals and an unpredictable economy that turns healthcare into a "luxury" for many Americans. Disparities exist in health status among various racial and ethnic groups and among those of differing socioeconomic status. Disparities exist in the use of health services and even in the types of treatment that are provided individuals in different social categories.

The first decade of the twenty-first century is also witnessing a further reaction to managed care. Capitated reimbursement arrangements are becoming less common, the gatekeeper concept is being abandoned, and consumer choice is being reintroduced into the market. Baby boomers are increasingly driving the market, shaping patterns of utilization and creating a demand for new services. At the same time, the growing population of elderly Americans is creating a demand for senior services far greater than anything ever experienced in the past.

Information technology is an increasingly important force shaping healthcare. The new healthcare calls for effective information management and data analysis. The demands of the Health Insurance Portability and Accountability Act (HIPAA) are bringing information technology issues to the forefront. This is being accompanied by the rise of e-health, perhaps the most significant development in healthcare in several years. The use of the Internet in the distribution of health information, the servicing of patients and plan enrollees, and the distribution of healthcare products promises to significantly change relationships within the healthcare arena.

THE ORGANIZATION OF U.S. HEALTH CARE

Healthcare is one of the more complex components of U.S. society. Its complexity is such that it is hard to define and even more difficult to describe in meaningful terms. Is healthcare an industry? A system? An institution? In actuality, it is all of these and more. As shall be seen, much of what healthcare is depends on one's perspective, although the sections that follow will be viewed within an institutional context. Not surprisingly, one's perception of the nature of healthcare has important implications for the approach to communication.

An encyclopedia would be required to fully describe the multiple dimensions of American healthcare, and that is certainly not appropriate here. The material that follows is restricted to the information necessary to appreciate the healthcare system relative to the field of health communication. While some will no doubt be critical of what has been included and excluded, the author has made his best effort to restrict this material to that relevant within the context of the remainder of this book.

A useful starting point for attempting to examine the organization of U.S. healthcare would be to inventory its component parts. The U.S. healthcare system has an incredible number of functioning units, including approximately 6,400 hospitals, over 15,000 nursing homes, and an estimated 300,000 clinics providing physician care. These figures do not include nonphysician providers and other personnel such as chiropractors and mental health counselors.

The "providers" of care typically are autonomous parties operating under a variety of guises and means of control. Healthcare providers—whether facilities or practitioners—can be organized as private for-profit organizations, private not-for-profit organizations, public organizations, and quasi-public organizations, among others. Similarly, they may be owned by private investors, publicly held, local-government owned and operated, or run by a religious denomination, foundation, or some other nonprofit entity.

The complexity of the U.S. healthcare system is reflected in the proliferation of occupational roles, the levels and stages of care that are provided (along both vertical and horizontal continua), and the almost unlimited points at which a patient might enter the system. The end result, many observers contend, is a "non-system" that is poorly integrated, lacks centralized control and regulation, and is characterized by fragmentation, discontinuity, and duplication.

The Structure of Healthcare

A useful approach to understanding the healthcare system is to conceptualize it in terms of *levels* of care. These levels are generally referred to as primary care, secondary care, and tertiary care. Additionally, some observers have identified a fourth category—quaternary care—to be applied to superspecialized services such as organ transplantation and trauma care. These levels can be viewed as the vertical dimension of the healthcare delivery system.

Primary care refers to the provision of the most basic health services. These generally involve the care of minor, routine problems, along with the provision of general examinations and preventive services. For the patient, primary care usually involves some self-care, perhaps followed by the seeking of care from a non-physician health professional such as a pharmacist. For certain ethnic groups, this may involve the use of a "folk" healer.

Formal primary care services are generally provided by physicians with training in general or family practice, general internal medicine, obstetrics/gynecology, and pediatrics. These practitioners are typically community based (rather than hospital based), rely on direct first contact with patients rather than receiving referrals from other physicians, and provide continuous rather than episodic care. Physician extenders like nurse practitioners and physician assistants are taking on a growing responsibility for primary care. In the mental health system, psychologists and other types of counselors constitute the primary level of care. Medical specialists provide a certain amount of primary care.

Primary care is generally delivered at the physician's office or at some type of clinic. Hospital outpatient departments, urgent care centers, freestanding surgery centers, and other ambulatory care facilities also provide primary care services. For certain segments of the population, the hospital emergency room serves as a source of primary care. The home has increasingly become a site of choice for the provision of primary care. This trend has been driven by a number of factors, including financial pressures on inpatient care, changing consumer preferences, and improved home care technology.

In terms of hospital services, primary care refers to those services that can be provided at a "general" hospital. These typically involve routine medical and surgical procedures, diagnostic tests, and obstetrical services. Primary care also includes basic emergency care (although not major trauma) and many outpatient services. Primary hospital care tends to be unspecialized and requires a relatively low level of technological sophistication. In actuality, there are few remaining hospitals that could truly be considered to provide "primary care". Even the smallest hospital today is likely to have equipment that may not have been available in major hospitals only a few years ago.

Secondary care reflects a higher degree of specialization and technological sophistication than primary care. Physician care is provided by more highly trained practitioners such as specialized surgeons (e.g., urologists and ophthalmologists) and specialized internists (e.g., cardiologists and oncologists). Problems requiring more specialized skills and more sophisticated biomedical equipment fall into this category. Although much of the care is still provided in the physician office or clinic, these specialists tend to spend a larger share of their time in the hospital setting. Secondary hospitals are capable of providing more complex technological backup, physician specialist support, and ancillary services than primary care hospitals. These facilities are capable of handling moderately complex surgical and medical cases and serve as referral centers for primary care facilities.

Tertiary care addresses the more complex of surgical and medical conditions. The practitioners tend to be subspecialists and the facilities highly complex and technologically advanced. Complex procedures such as open-heart surgery, and reconstructive surgery are performed at these facilities, which provide extensive support services in terms of both personnel and technology. Tertiary care cases are usually handled by a team of medical and/or surgical specialists who are supported by the hospital's radiology, pathology, and anesthesiology physician staff. Tertiary care is generally provided at a few centers that serve large geographical areas. Frequently, a single hospital is not sufficient for the provision of tertiary care; a "medical center" may be required. These centers typically support functions not directly related to patient care, such as teaching and research.

Some procedures often performed at tertiary facilities may be considered as *quaternary care*. Organ transplantation—especially involving vital organs like heart, lungs and pancreas—and complicated trauma cases are examples. This level of care is restricted to major medical centers often in medical school settings. These procedures require the most sophisticated equipment and are often performed in association with research activities.

THE EVOLVING HEALTHCARE ENVIRONMENT

During the last two decades of the twentieth century the U.S. health-care system underwent a major transformation. The changes that have taken place in healthcare have been numerous and dramatic. These changes have served to transform the healthcare industry of the early 1980s into a quite different institution entering the twenty-first century. These changes, as it turns out, also have had significant implications for health communication. Space does not allow a review of all of the changes that occurred during the last decade and a half, but some of the more important ones are listed below, along with their significance for health communication.

The environment for communicating about health has changed significantly over past years, and it will no doubt continue to change in the future. These changes include dramatic increases in the number of communication channels and the number of health issues vying for public attention. They include increasing consumer demands for more and better quality health information. And they include increasing sophistication of marketing and sales techniques, such as direct-to-consumer advertising of prescription drugs and sales of medical devices and medications over the Internet. The growing prominence of health issues on the public agenda increases competition for people's time and attention; at the same time, people have more opportunities to select information based on their personal interests and preferences because of increased communication channels. The trend toward commercialization of the Internet suggests that the marketing model of other mass media will be applied to these emerging media, which has important consequences for the ability of noncommercial and public health-oriented health communication to stand out in a cluttered health information environment.

Although the 1950s was viewed as the "marketing era" outside of healthcare, the more aggressive promotional techniques characterizing other industries were essentially not on the radar screen in healthcare during this decade. True, the emerging pharmaceutical industry was beginning to market to physicians and the fledging insurance industry was beginning to market health plans. In the healthcare trenches, however, healthcare providers were light-years away from formal marketing activities. Hospitals and physicians, for the most part, considered formal promotional activities to be inappropriate and even unethical. Marketing on the part of hospitals did occur through free educational programs and public relations activities. Even as the hospital industry came of age and large numbers of new facilities were established, the industry continued to reflect a traditional approach to communication.

As the health services sector expanded during the 1960s, the role of public relations was enhanced. While the developments that would eventually force hospitals and other healthcare organizations to embrace formal marketing techniques were at least a decade away, the field of public relations was flourishing. This communication function remained the healthcare organization's primary means of keeping in touch with its various publics—especially the physicians who admitted or referred patients to their facilities and the donors who made charitable contributions to the organization. Consumers were not considered an important constituency, since they did not directly choose hospitals but were referred by their physicians or steered by their health plans. The use of media to advance strategic marketing objectives had not evolved, and media relations in this era often consisted of answering reporters' questions about patient conditions.

Print was the medium of choice for communication throughout the 1960s in spite of the increasingly influential role that the electronic media were playing for marketers in other industries. This was the era of polished annual reports, informational brochures, and publications targeted to the community. Health communication became a well-developed function, and hospitals continued to expand their public relations activity.

The 1970s witnessed the growing importance of the for-profit hospital sector. During this decade, a growing urgency appeared among hospitals with regard to taking their case to the community. This was coupled with the growing conviction that, in the future, healthcare organizations were going to have to be able to attract patients. Legal restrictions on marketing were loosened, and many organizations extended their public relations functions to include a broader marketing mandate. The increased interest in health communication of all forms spurred more formalization in the field.

By the 1970s, hospitals were recognizing the role that patients might play in the hospital selection decision. In the mid-1970s, many hospitals adopted mass advertising strategies to promote their programs, including the use of billboard displays and television and radio commercials touting the facility. The advertising goal was to encourage patients to use the hospital facilities when the doctor presented a choice, or to self-refer if necessary (Berkowitz 1996).

Competition for patients was increasing, and hospitals and other providers with limited experience in more formal marketing techniques turned to the familiar function of public relations in their promotional efforts. Communication efforts were beginning to be targeted toward patients, and patient satisfaction research grew in importance.

Health communication activity exploded in 1980s as marketing became an increasingly accepted function for healthcare organizations. Employers and consumers had become key purchasers of healthcare, and the physician's role in referring patients for hospital services was beginning to diminish. The dramatic growth of mega-chains of hospitals and other facilities was initiated during this period, and this development was to have a profound effect on communication requirements. Further, hospitals realized that by taking their message directly to consumers for services such as obstetrics, cosmetic surgery, and outpatient care, they could generate revenue and enhance market share.

Although marketing was beginning to be accepted, healthcare suffered from a lack of professional marketing personnel. While traditional approaches to health communication were well developed, few health professionals were experienced with more formal marketing techniques. It became necessary to turn to outside resources for the development of more aggressive communication campaigns.

The rise of service line marketing launched the great hospital advertising wars of the 1980s. Barely a blip on the healthcare marketing radar screen a decade earlier, the growth of advertising during this decade was dramatic. The proliferation of hospital advertising was fueled by an increasingly competitive marketplace and a belief among marketing professionals that advertising was the key to competitive success. Once a medium of dubious respectability, advertising was now hailed as a marketing panacea for hospitals (Berkowitz 1996).

During this period, marketing came to be seen as the most important form of health communication and advertising as the most important form of marketing. Ultimately, this surge in advertising was both a blessing and a curse. Advertising campaigns were something relatively concrete that the organization could invest in. Establishing advertising budgets and developing advertising initiatives was the quickest way to get marketing incorporated into healthcare and to gain some visibility for this function. On the other hand, the lack of success of much healthcare advertising and the often negative fallout it generated were definitely setbacks for health communication.

By the 1980s, managed care was becoming a major force in healthcare and this would have important implications for health communication. As managed care penetration increased, the plan member—rather than the patient—became the target for communication. This resulted in an important shift in the goal of communication. Communication no longer focused primarily on information dissemination, but on the more challenging task of developing relationships. For managed care to work, plan members had to be well informed and encouraged to follow certain practices. Even if they never became ill, they still required communication.

As healthcare became market-driven in the 1990s, the communication function grew in importance within healthcare organizations. The institutional perspective that had long driven decision making gave way to market-driven decision making. Everything was now being looked at from the point of view of customers and other external audiences. The popularity of guest relations programs during the 1990s solidified the transformation of "patients" into "customers". Every hospital was now trying to win the "hearts and minds" battle for the healthcare consumer.

The mergers and consolidation that took place during this decade resulted in the creation of larger organizations that had more resources and more sophisticated management. Executives entered the field from outside of healthcare, bringing a more businesslike atmosphere. Public relations achieved new status as the "positioning" tool of choice. To gain credibility for newly merged health systems or to reinforce positioning for established ones, healthcare organizations turned to various print and electronic media. The media relations function became a strategic tool for showcasing clinical centers of excellence or institutional programs. The rise in health care media and the interactive technology of the Internet combined to create an "informed consumer" who is more empowered with information than at any time in human history.

The consumer was rediscovered during this process, and the direct-to-consumer movement was an outgrowth of these developments. As consumers gained in influence, marketing became increasingly integrated into the operations of healthcare organizations. The consumers of the 1990s were better educated and more assertive about their healthcare needs than consumers of a generation ago. The emergence of the Internet as a source of health information furthered the rise of consumerism. Newly empowered consumers were taking on an increasingly influential, if informal, role in reshaping the American health care system. Consumers were beginning to challenge physicians and their health plans armed with unprecedented knowledge.

Accountability became a hallmark of the new consumerism and was evidenced by the "report cards" issued by health plans and healthcare providers. Increasingly, employer groups and consumers were beginning to demand measurable clinical outcomes data on providers and health plans. Empowered consumers demanded information on the services and pricing for health plans, hospitals, and physicians as they sought to make informed decisions. The backlash against managed care along with consumer's rights legislation further improved the standing of the consumer.

Consumer research grew in importance during this decade. The need for information on consumers, customers, competitors and the market demanded expansion of the research function. Patient and consumer research was augmented and newly developed technologies brought the research capabilities of other industries to healthcare.

The context for health communication as we enter a new millennium continues to evolve. In the 1990s, the emphasis shifted from sick people to well people in response to the emergence of managed care and capitated payments. There was a new focus on patient satisfaction and increased efforts toward generating consumer data. The baby boomers who were coming to dominate the healthcare landscape were hungry for information. Techniques from other industries, like customer relationship marketing, began receiving attention.

With the repackaging and maturation of marketing in the 1990s, the health communication field became more sophisticated overall. The market was in many ways more competitive and even the managed care environment held opportunities for promotional activities. In addition, the mergers that occurred not only created more potential marketing clout, but often involved for-profit healthcare organizations that were inherently more marketing oriented.

The trend of rapidly expanding opportunities in health communication intersects with recent demands for more rigorous evaluation of all aspects of the health care and public health delivery systems and for evidence-based practices. There is growing research on the process of health information-seeking and the role of health information in decision making. Health communication campaigns are benefiting from more rigorous formative research and evaluation of outcomes.

HEALTHCARE DEVELOPMENTS

There are a number of developments that have affected healthcare during recent years and most continue to play a role going into the 21st century. Some of the major developments that are affecting healthcare and, hence, the field of health communication are described below.

Growing Competition Among Healthcare Organizations

During the 1980s, healthcare providers were exposed to unprecedented competition on a number of fronts. For the first time, healthcare providers were forced to profile their customers and be able to determine their needs. They also had to understand their competition and develop a level of market intelligence never dreamed of in the past. Healthcare providers were faced with the challenge of communicating—efficiently and effectively—with both existing patients and potential clients, many of them for the first time.

The Shift from Inpatient Care to Outpatient Care

Until the last decade or so of the twentieth century, medical care was synonymous with inpatient care. Hospitalization was often a prerequisite for the activation of insurance coverage. By the 1980s, almost every industry force was discouraging the use of inpatient care. Hospitals had to rapidly understand changing market conditions and position themselves to capture the growing outpatient market. Hospitals had to think in terms of a different approach for communicating with their constituents as the traditional patterns of physician referral for inpatient care were de-emphasized and consumerism emerged as a factor in the system. The shift to outpatient care resulted in more consumer choice which, in turn, meant that more communication with consumers was required.

The Shift from Specialty Care to Primary Care

Hospitals have historically relied upon the medical specialists on their staffs to admit patients and generate their revenue. By the late 1980s, industry forces were encouraging the use of primary care physicians rather than specialists. Hospital systems had to examine their referral patterns and revise their thinking with regard to primary care physicians. For the first time, hospitals had to actively court family practitioners, internists and pediatricians, and marketers had to develop means for showcasing their primary care capabilities to both consumers and health plans.

Employers as a Major Force

After World War II, employers began offering health insurance to their employees and passively footed the bill for their medical expenses. By the mid-1980s, however, employers were taking a more active role in the management of their employees' health benefits. Suddenly, healthcare providers found they had a new customer with a different set of needs from their traditional customers. Business coalitions emerged to negotiate with healthcare providers from a position of strength. Employers found it important to communicate more aggressively with their employees on health issues, on the one hand, providing them relevant health information and, on the other, receiving feedback from them on the care they receive. Health plans had to become better communicators to employers if they hoped to retain their contracts.

The Market as a Driving Force

Until the healthcare industry became market driven in the 1980s, the opinions of patients were seldom considered important. All of a sudden, healthcare providers needed to know what the patient liked and did not like about the services provided. Patient satisfaction surveys became commonplace, and various groups started issuing "report cards" that rated the performance of providers and health plans. Marketers were called upon to not only identify the wants and needs of the market, but to assist in maintaining a high level of customer satisfaction. The major shift from a production orientation to a market orientation on the part of healthcare providers now meant that the market was driving the bus. This invariably resulted in stepped-up communication with the consumers who constituted the market.

Managed Care as a Dominant Force

The emergence of managed care as a major force essentially changed the ground rules for healthcare providers. The patient was now transformed into an enrollee. Instead of searching for sick patients that would require health services, it became important to identify healthy persons that would not consume very many services. Healthcare providers participating in managed care plans (particularly capitated plans) had to shift their focus from treatment and cure to health maintenance. Managed care plans had to develop marketing expertise in order to capture the employer market, and managed care negotiations came to be considered a marketing function by many health systems. Under managed care, it was to the advantage of health plans to communicate often and extensively with their enrollees in order to effect the changes required to "manage" their care. "Doctor's orders" were increasingly replaced by the more persuasive approach embodied by health communication.

The Changing Decision Maker

In the pre-marketing era in healthcare, virtually all decisions were made by physicians, and consumers had limited control over their medical episodes. Later, health plans began exercising inordinate influence over the use of health services as their enrollees were directed to specific provider networks. During the 1990s, consumers began to wield considerable influence as consumer-choice began to characterize the industry, and the prospect of "defined contributions" brought a new perspective to health communication. Pharmaceutical companies and health plans, who had traditionally marketed to "middlemen", were now communicating directly with the consumer. Despite the impact of managed care, many of the developments of the late 20th century served to atomize the healthcare market, thereby complicating the task of those in health communication.

Redefining the "Patient"

Of all of the developments in healthcare of the past two or three decades, perhaps the one with the most implications for health communication is the redefining of the patient. By the end of the twentieth century, the term "patient" was being replaced by "client", "customer", "consumer", or "enrollee", depending on the situation. The major consideration regardless of the label was the fact that clients, customers, consumers and enrollees all had different characteristics than did patients. While the term "patient" implies a dependent, submissive status, each of these other terms implies that the party so labeled is more proactively involved in the provision of his or her care. Healthcare "consumers" (that is, patients with the attitudes of customers) were spawned by the Baby Boom generation and are used to higher level of service than that typically offered through the healthcare system. They are demanding more attention from practitioners and more of a partnership in the therapeutic process. Ultimately, this development influenced the manner in which the various players in healthcare interact and transformed the context for health communication.

The redefinition of the patient has had major implications for health communication. Communicating with a consumer is not the same as communicating with a patient, with modifications required in the message and the medium. The source of information is less likely to be the physician and more likely to represent a more impersonal source such as direct mail or the Internet. One advantage of this shift is the availability of a wide range of promotional techniques that are appropriate for consumers or customers but not for patients. (Box 3.1 discusses the shifts in sources of health information that have been occurring.)

Box 3.1

New Sources of Health Information

Traditionally, healthcare consumers have had access to two primary sources of information on healthcare—one informal and one formal. The primary source of health information historically has been friends, relatives, neighbors and work associates, individuals who can be informally accessed for information. Thus, based on their own experiences and information they have gathered, these associates could offer insights into various providers and services. The formal source that may be somewhat less common but more authoritative is physicians and other health personnel. By virtue of their position within the system and their presumed knowledge, doctors in particular have been a major source of information on healthcare.

Box 3.1 (Continued).

These two major sources are being supplemented by information gleaned from the media. This has historically included news obtained from print media (e.g., magazines and newspapers) and electronic media (e.g., radio and television). Newsletters geared to the needs of healthcare consumers have become common and, of course, there is no end to the number and variety of self-help books published for those seeking health information.

These two sources of knowledge continue to be important to healthcare consumers today, but they have begun sharing space with other sources of information. With the introduction of Medicare and Medicaid in the 1960s and the emergence of managed care in the 1980s, healthcare consumers have been increasingly turning to their health plans in search of information on healthcare providers. This development reflects to a great extent the restrictions on the use of practitioners, facilities and programs imposed by the health plans. But it also indicates the growing importance of health plans as a valuable source of information on the system. Managed care plans have been particularly aggressive in establishing call centers and encouraging their enrollees to seek information prior to any health-related decisions.

The other source of healthcare information that really came to the fore in the 1990s was the World Wide Web. The Internet has become a major source of health-related information, and there are purportedly more sites in cyberspace related to health than any other topic. A majority of "wired" healthcare consumers has accessed the Internet for information on a health issue they or someone else faced. Consumers are increasingly armed with Internet-generated information when they present themselves at the doctor's office. While the quality of the available data and the implications for medical practice of better-informed patients certainly merit discussion, it is clear that the World Wide Web is replacing more traditional sources as the first resort in healthcare consumer information search.

References

Berkowitz, Eric N. (1996). *Essentials of health care marketing*. Gaithersburg, MD: Aspen Publishers.

Engle, George L. (1977). The need for a new medical model: A challenge for bioscience. *Science*, 196, 129–135.

Omran, A.R. (1971). The epidemiologic transition: A theory of the epidemiology of population change. *Milbank Memorial Fund Quarterly*, 49, 515ff.

Chapter 4
The History of Health Communication

C hapter 4 presents a brief history of the field of health communication, beginning with background on the evolution of communication in general and then focusing on the emergence of health communication as a separate field. The factors involved in the evolution of health communication are reviewed and its roots in other disciplines are discussed. The current state of knowledge on the field of health communication is reviewed and gaps in our knowledge on this topic noted.

The emergence of health as an important personal concern and the ascendancy of healthcare as a major institution in the middle of the 20th century in the U.S. were major factors in the evolution of the field of health communication. The conceptualization of "health" as a distinct value in U.S. society represented a major development in the emergence of the healthcare institution. Prior to World War II health was generally not recognized as a value by Americans but was vaguely tied in with other notions of well-being. In the decades following the war personal health became a growing concern, and the adequate provision of health services became an important issue in the mind of the American public. By the last third of the twentieth century, health had become an obsession with Americans.

Once health became established as a value, it was a short step to establishing a formal healthcare system as the institutional means for achieving that value. An environment was created that encouraged the emergence of a powerful institution that supported many other contemporary American values. In the second half of the 20th century emerging American values combined to give impetus to the growth of the industry. The value that Americans came to place on youth, beauty and self-actualization further contributed to an expansion of the role of healthcare. The ability of the nascent healthcare system to address emerging U.S. values and garner support from the economic, political, and educational institutions assured the ascendancy of this new institutional form.

EARLY EFFORTS AT HEALTH COMMUNICATION

During the early days of medicine in a fledging America, health communication in a formal sense was poorly developed. The field of communication was not recognized as a distinct discipline and much was accorded to the arena of "common sense". To be sure, there were announcements of quarantine and other communications related to contagious diseases. But the formal application of health communication was a long way off.

Prior to the emergence of modern medicine, health communication was primarily informal. The practitioners of folk medicine—which was virtually everyone—communicated the ingredients, techniques and lore surrounding the use of natural materials for the management of disease and injury. Intergenerational communication was critical in the passing on of the accumulated knowledge of folk medicine to subsequent generations.

Even in the early twentieth century few people had occasion to use doctors. Few physicians were available, and those that were lacked the type of training we take for granted today. There was no dominant medical paradigm and, in a democratic society, any man's medicine was as good as the next one's. In actually, those who passed for "doctors" in those days had little in the way of knowledge, tools, or skills when it came to most of the conditions that existed within the population. The one tool they did have, however, was their communication skills—their bedside manner, if you will—that they developed during the course of their careers. Given the fact that no one had the necessary skills to cure most diseases, medical historians report that those with effective communication skills had the best chance of affecting a cure.

Today we recognize the importance of a healing environment and the impact that communication can have on the course of an illness. We have empirically demonstrated what many early doctors no doubt knew intuitively: the mind and body are closely connected, and one's social context has important implications for one's health.

FACTORS AFFECTING THE EVOLUTION
OF HEALTH COMMUNICATION

The New Medical Model

The formulation of the germ theory with the subsequent emergence of the allopathic model as *the* approach to healthcare was a mixed blessing. There is no need to catalogue here the impact of the then-new medical model on the diagnosis and treatment of many health conditions. While the contribution of scientific medicine to the conquest of disease is perhaps overstated in the popular mind (McKinley and McKinley, 1977), an approach to the management of illness was created that contributed to greatly improved health status for individuals and communities.

The downside of the ascendancy of the medical model was the setback that it caused health communication. As the field became more science-based, it became increasingly reductionist, with all health problems pursued down to the lowest level—from the person to the body system to the organ to the cellular structure. With each successive step, the patient as a whole person receded further into the background.

The direct implication of this development was the demeaning of the importance of communication. Bedside manner was relegated to the medical archives, since the answer to the problem was to be found under the microscope and not within the patient. While some physicians developed an effective bedside manner, organized medicine came to see this as an unnecessary skill.

During the "golden age" of medicine in the United States—the 1960s and 70s—health communication was further pushed to the background. As medicine became more scientific, the importance of detached objectivity came to the fore. Rather than coming to understand the totality of the patient, physicians were now trained to remain distant and uninvolved, lest personal feelings interfere with the march of medical progress.

Since it was impossible to totally avoid communication with patients and/or their families, the conversation of physicians became filled with medical jargon. Their new-found scientific knowledge allowed them to demonstrate the level of skill they possessed and created a clear separation between the learned practitioner and the ignorant patient. Thus, physicians came to use scientific terminology that they were reluctant to explain to patients. Further, the asymmetric nature of the relationship discouraged questions on the part of patients—lest they appear to question the pronouncements of the good doctor. These developments contributed to a decline in the quality of doctor-patient interaction.

The Rise of Consumerism

By the end of the 1970s, a reaction to this approach to doctor-patient relationships had emerged. Some refer to it as the "patient education movement"; others see it within a broader context of "consumerism" that affected other institutions in the society besides healthcare. This movement partly reflected the growth in knowledge about the nature of the healthcare system and its effectiveness, and contributed to the mounting criticism of the healthcare system and its operation. The consumer movement found that patients in particular and healthcare consumers in general were woefully ignorant of the nature of health and illness and unable to contribute to their health status in a meaningful way.

The causes for this failure of communication have been attributed primarily to the healthcare system and particularly on its pivotal practitioner, the physician. Observers cited the deliberate efforts on the part of physicians to hamper communication, deter the transfer of knowledge, and obscure the situation in the mind of the patient. Practitioners justified their lapses in communication on the grounds that patients were unable to intelligently talk about their problems, a claim that was refuted by research indicating reasonable knowledge on the part of patients, even patients considered to be disadvantaged.

Discrimination in Healthcare

These developments occurred within a context of growing concerns about many aspects of society. While it was acknowledged that certain groups in U.S. society were discriminated against in terms of jobs, education, housing and other benefits of society, it became increasingly clear that the healthcare system was also discriminatory with regard to many groups within society. While medical practitioners related well to well-educated, affluent patients who could more or less "speak their language", they did not relate at all well to minority populations or those from different socioeconomic backgrounds.

The differences found in the communication modalities of medical professionals has contributed to the now well-documented disparities between various groups in society with regard to health status, health behavior and the manner of treatment received.

Growing Emphasis on Prevention

Another emerging trend over the last quarter of the 20th century has been the realization that prevention could potentially play a greater role in the improvement of health status than treatment could. This led to the realization that the standard approach—repairing broken bodies—was not as effective in improving health status as preventive measures were. A growing body of research on the potential of preventive measures has served to boost this dimension of healthcare and dampened our enthusiasm for the more aggressive aspects of treatment and cure.

The rise of consumerism occurred within the context of a major shift in attitudes within the population. The Baby Boom generation was coming of age and developed characteristics unlike those of any previous generation. This population was much more proactive than previous generations and craved communication on health issues.

The Acceptance of Marketing by Healthcare

One of the major contributors to the emergence of formal health communication was the incorporation of marketing into the healthcare system. Health communication could be thought of as a subdivision of marketing in some senses, although there are many aspects of health communication that are not designed to promote an idea, organization or product. The field of health communication has clearly benefited from the emergence of marketing in healthcare. This development has led to stepped up efforts in consumer research, a better understanding of the communication process, and access to more effective communication techniques, among other benefits.

The rise of marketing in healthcare has also contributed to the emergence of social marketing as an approach to health communication. Social marketing makes use of many of the techniques that have been developed to reach consumers in other industries and takes advantage of contemporary approaches to information dissemination.

THE GROWTH OF HEALTH COMMUNICATION

Although the 1950s is considered to mark the beginning of the "marketing era" in the United States, the establishment of the marketing function within the U.S. economy took several decades, and marketers had to overcome a number of factors that retarded its development (Thomas, 2004). Newly empowered consumers demanded a growing array of goods and services, even if existing goods and services had adequately served previous generations. A growing consumer market with expanding needs, coupled with a proliferation of products, created an unprecedented demand for consumer information.

Healthcare adopted marketing approaches well after most other industries, and the marketing era was not considered to begin in healthcare until the 1980s. Pharmaceutical companies, consumer products vendors, and health plans have a long history of marketing activities; indeed, some of these organizations devote an inordinate proportion of their budgets to marketing. While marketing was noticeably absent from the functions of most healthcare providers until the 1980s, precursors to marketing had long been established. Every hospital and many other healthcare organizations had well-established public relations (PR) functions. PR involved disseminating information concerning the organization and announcing new developments. The main interface for PR staff was with the media. They disseminated press releases, responded to requests for information, and served as the interface with the press should some negative event occur.

Large provider organizations typically established communications departments for developing materials for dissemination to the public and the employees of the organization. Internal (and, later, patient-oriented) newsletters and patient education materials were frequently developed by communications staff. Some of the larger organizations (and certainly the major retail firms and professional associations) established government relations offices. They served as the interface with government officials and provided lobbying efforts as appropriate.

In addition to these formal precursors of marketing, healthcare organizations of all types were involved in informal communication activities to a certain extent. This occurred when hospitals sponsored health education seminars, held an open house for a new facility, or supported a community event. Hospitals marketed themselves by making their facilities available to the community for public meetings and otherwise attempting to be good corporate citizens. Physicians marketed themselves through networking with their colleagues at the country club or medical society–sponsored events. All of these activities relied on effective communication.

Print was the medium of choice for communication throughout the 1960s, in spite of the increasingly influential role the electronic media were playing for marketers in other industries. This was the era of polished annual reports, informational brochures, and publications targeted to the community. Health communication became a well-developed function, and hospitals continued to expand their PR function.

During the 1970s, hospitals felt a growing urgency to take their case to the community. This was coupled with the growing conviction that, in the future, healthcare organizations were going to have to be able to attract patients. Legal restrictions on marketing were loosened, and many organizations extended their PR functions to include a broader marketing mandate. Such activity appeared to be particularly strong in parts of the country where health maintenance organizations (HMOs) were emerging. Competition for patients was increasing, and hospitals and other providers turned to the familiar PR function for their promotional efforts. Communication efforts were beginning to be targeted toward patients, and patient satisfaction research grew in importance.

Health communicators had to begin looking at audiences in an entirely different way, and the importance of consumers was heightened by the introduction of the prospective payment system. Hospitals began to think of medical care in terms of product or service lines, a development that was to have major consequences for the marketing of health services. Hospitals realized the benefits derived from communicating directly to consumers for services such as obstetrics, cosmetic surgery, and outpatient care.

The proliferation of hospital advertising was fueled by an increasingly competitive marketplace and a belief among marketing professionals that advertising was the key to competitive success. Whatever the problem, advertising was viewed as the solution. In fact, many marketing directors defined their marketing programs in terms of the size of their advertising budget. However, much of the advertising of the mid to late 1980s was ineffectual at best and disastrous at worst. Many of the campaigns involved poorly conceived strategies and led to an enormous waste of dollars.

As healthcare became market driven in the 1990s, the communication function grew in importance within healthcare organizations. The institutional perspective that had long driven decision making gave way to market-driven decision making. Hospital policies and procedures that had been established for the convenience of the hospital staff, not for the benefit of the patient, were reexamined from the point of view of customers and other external audiences. The popularity of guest relations programs during the 1990s solidified the transformation of *patients* into *customers*. The 1990s represented a turning point in developing a real marketing perspective in healthcare. Every hospital was now trying to win the "hearts and minds" battle for the healthcare consumer.

The consumer was rediscovered during this process, and the direct-to-consumer movement was an outgrowth of these developments. As consumers gained influence, marketing became increasingly integrated into the operations of healthcare organizations. The consumers of the 1990s were better educated and more assertive about their healthcare needs than consumers of the previous generation. The emergence of the Internet as a source of health information furthered the rise of consumerism. Newly empowered consumers were taking on an increasingly influential (if informal) role in reshaping the U.S. healthcare system. Armed with unprecedented knowledge, consumers were beginning to challenge the control of information maintained by physicians and health plans.

During the 1990s, health professionals developed a new appreciation of the benefits of communication. A more qualified corps of marketing professionals who brought ambitious but realistic expectations to the industry emerged. Pharmaceutical companies began advertising directly to consumers, and this development made everyone in the industry more aware of marketing. In addition, virtually everyone in healthcare was becoming more consumer sensitive, and data that allowed for a better understanding of the healthcare customer were becoming available.

The emergence of marketing as an accepted function in healthcare had several important implications for health communication. First, this development brought heightened attention to all types of "promotional" activities, including communication. Health professionals became sensitized to the need for meaningful, on-going communication with their employees, customers and constituents. Efforts to create marketing-oriented organizations called for the widespread dissemination of information.

Some might argue that the new emphasis on the more overt forms of promotions such as advertising, direct mail, and personal sales would relegate the communication effort to a back seat. This does not appear to have happened as health communication functions have continued to remain strong throughout the evolution of marketing in healthcare.

The more important consideration is the increased significance accorded to communication within the context of marketing. Regardless of the marketing technique utilized, the ultimate goal is to communicate. This is particularly true in healthcare given the nature of the system, its providers and its customers. Marketers supporting a wide range of promotional techniques were all faced with the challenge of communicating their message to the target audience. This brought attention to theories of communication, the communication process, and the techniques that were being utilized to communicate in other settings.

References

McKinley, John, & Sonja J. McKinley. (1977). The questionable contribution of medical measures to the decline of mortality in the united states in the twentieth century. *Milbank Memorial Fund Quarterly/Health and Society*, 405–428.

Thomas, Richard K. (2004). *Marketing health services*. Chicago: Health Administration Press.

Chapter 5

Health Communication Audiences

A critical early step in developing a health communication initiative is the identification and profiling of the target audience. The various potential audiences for health communication activities are described in this chapter and the implications of their respective attributes discussed. Differences in the characteristics of individuals (e.g., patients, caregivers), social groups (e.g., medical practice staff), and communities as audiences are reviewed.

THE VARIETY OF HEALTHCARE AUDIENCES

One of the more important attributes of healthcare audiences that should be obvious by now is their variety. As will be seen below, we can think in terms of individuals as consumers of healthcare goods and services. Yet, health professionals and facilities are also major consumers of goods and services in the healthcare arena. While the needs may be different for organizations than for individuals, many of the same communication issues remain.

Healthcare consumers fall into a variety of different categories, each with specific needs. We usually think of those requiring life-saving services as the typical patient. In actuality, these are rare occurrences, but, when they do occur, they require dedicated personnel, equipment and facilities for their management. A more common category of consumers includes those who require "routine" health services. These include the typical person who presents himself for treatment at a doctor's office, clinic, or therapy center. A third category includes consumers who desire elective health services. These include products and/or services that are considered discretionary or not considered "medically necessary".

47

There is also the major category of consumers who are involved in self-care. Research indicates that the amount of self-care is much greater than previously thought and that accessing the formal healthcare system typically occurs only *after* other options have been exhausted. Thus, it is typical for symptomatic individuals to self diagnose and self medicate, employing the wide range of "do-it-yourself" healthcare products that have become available. Pharmacy shelves have become stocked with a variety of products and devices for home testing and treatment, and the Internet has expanded the availability of such products.

For these and other reasons, a number of different terms are being applied today to the purchasers and/or end-users of healthcare goods and services. At the practitioner level, the term "patient" is giving way to other terms that more clearly reflect the contemporary healthcare environment. The major terms used to characterize health communication audiences are described below.

Consumers

"Consumer", as typically used in healthcare, refers to any individual or organization that is a potential purchaser of a healthcare product. (This differs from the more economics-based notion of consumer as the entity that actually *consumes* the product.) Theoretically, everyone is a potential consumer of health services, and consumer research often targets the public at large. The healthcare consumer is often the end-user of a good or service but may not necessarily be the purchaser. "Consumer behavior" refers to the utilization patterns and purchasing practices of the population of a market area.

Customers

The "customer" is typically thought of in healthcare as the actual purchaser of a good or service. While a patient may be a customer for certain goods and services, it is often the case that the end-user (e.g., the patient) may not be the customer. Someone else may make the purchase on behalf of the patient, and treatment decisions may be made by someone other than the patient.

For this reason, hospitals and other complex healthcare organizations are likely to serve a range of customers. These may include patients, staff physicians, health plans, employers and a variety of other parties who may purchase goods or services from the organization. For this reason, the customer identification process in healthcare is more complicated than it is in other industries.

Clients

A client is a type of customer that consumes services rather than goods. A client relationship implies personal (rather than impersonal) interaction and an on-going relationship (rather than an episodic one). Professionals typically have clients while retailers, for example, would have customers or purchasers. A client is likely to have a more symmetrical relationship with a service provider than a patient who is typically dependent upon and powerless relative to the service provider. Many also feel that the term "client" implies more respect than the term "patient".

Patients

While the term "patient" is used rather loosely in informal discussion, a patient is technically someone who has been admitted into the formal system of healthcare. A prerequisite for this status is the defining of the individual as "sick" by a physician. Technically, a symptomatic individual does not become a patient until a physician officially designates the individual as such, even if he has consumed over-the-counter drugs or taken other measures for self-care. Under this scenario, an individual remains a patient until he is discharged from medical care.

While non-physician clinicians may treat patients, it is often not considered appropriate for them to use that term. For example, mental health therapists are likely to refer to the people they provide services to as "clients" rather than "patients". Dependent practitioners who work under the supervision of physicians (e.g., physical therapists), however, are likely to define their charges as patients.

Enrollees

While health insurance plans have historically conceptualized their customers as "enrollees", this is a concept that has only recently become common among healthcare providers. However, with the ascendancy of managed care as a major force in healthcare, other healthcare organizations have begun to adopt this term. Thus, providers who contracted to provide services for members of a health plan began to think in terms of enrollees. This is a significant shift in nomenclature, since an enrollee has different attributes from a patient. The most important difference is the fact that a relationship is established with the individual *before* the onset of an illness episode, rather than once the person becomes ill. Further, the relationship with the enrolled extends beyond the end of the illness episode. Enrollees may be variously referred to as "members," "insureds," or "covered lives."

End-users

The ultimate consumer of health services, as in other industries, is referred to here as the "end-user", and all of the terms above may be used variously to refer to the end-user of health services. This term is typically not used by health professionals other than marketers. In healthcare, the end-user is typically the patient who is the direct recipient of a health service or the eventual consumer of a health product or over-the-counter drug. The end-user could also take the form of a health plan enrollee who eventually files claims for compensation for medical care.

The healthcare situation is unique in that the end-user may not play an active role in the selection of the goods or services to be consumed and is often insulated from the cost of these goods and services. A symptomatic individual may choose a physician (but most likely from a limited list of providers) or be assigned a physician as in the case of a Medicaid managed care plan. Once in the system, the end-user has limited options in terms of the direction of the care. The physician, the hospital staff, case managers, and other parties make most of the decisions for the consumer of the services. In many cases, the patient's family may provide input into the decision-making process. Even such important issues as whether to discontinue life-support may be made by someone other than the end-user.

PROFESSIONAL AND INSTITUTIONAL AUDIENCES

As noted above, the end-user of healthcare goods and services represents only one type of audience found in healthcare. Much of the consumption of goods and services is carried out by health professionals and healthcare institutions that may be viewed by many as customers. Although the *physician* is thought of as a provider of services rather than a consumer of them, physician practices may be viewed as customers by many other parties. Hospitals solicit physicians to join their medical staffs (and service them once they join). Provider networks and health plans solicit the participation of physicians and other clinicians. Nursing homes, home health agencies, and hospices may depend on them for their referrals. Many physicians depend on referrals from other physicians and those referring physicians represent customers.

Physicians also serve as customers for a variety of organizations providing support services. These include billing and collection services, utilization review companies, medical supply distributors, biomedical equipment companies, and biohazard management companies. Physicians are also customers for information technology vendors who sell and/or service practice management systems, imaging systems, and/or electronic patient records.

Physicians have traditionally been the primary target audience for pharmaceutical companies. The extent to which pharmaceutical companies will go to acquire physician loyalty to their drug lines is legendary. In fact, the sales and promotions efforts of pharmaceutical companies toward physicians became so intense that Congress ultimately had to pass regulations restricting attempts by pharmaceutical companies to influence the prescribing practices of physicians.

Other clinicians are customers for many of the same goods and services as physicians. Dentists, optometrists, podiatrists, chiropractors, mental health counselors and other independent practitioners have many of the same needs as physicians and are cultivated by similar marketing entities. These providers require supplies, equipment, billing and collections, information technology and other services just as physicians do. Since these practitioners typically cannot prescribe drugs, their business is not solicited by pharmaceutical companies.

Hospitals and other healthcare institutional settings have a wide-range of health-related requirements as well as the normal needs that any large organization must address. Like physicians, they require medical supplies and biomedical equipment. More so than physicians, they require durable medical equipment such as wheelchairs and hospital beds. They are customers for a wide range of support services, from billing and collections to physician recruitment to marketing. By virtue of providing food service, gift shops, and parking services, hospitals are customers for a wide variety of non-health related goods and services. Hospitals and other healthcare facilities are heavy consumers of information technology and are major customers for IT venders and consultants.

Major *employers* represent target audiences for health plans, managed care plans, providers and provider networks. Most health plans are employer-based, and competing health plans seek to contract with employers for the management of their employees' health. Individual providers may seek to contract with employers that are self-insured or otherwise open to negotiated services. Employers are also customers for a variety of direct services from providers. These include a wide range of occupational health services, employee assistance programs, fitness center programs, and various other services that providers might market directly to employers.

OTHER AUDIENCES

Like organizations in other industries, healthcare organizations have various "internal" audiences. Chief among these are their *employees*. Any organization must consider its workforce as a customer and healthcare organizations have, unfortunately, not been in the forefront in this regard. It is important to continuously "market" the mission, goals and objectives of the organization to these internal customers and to regularly solicit their input. Poor internal communications has been blamed for many of the dysfunctional aspects of healthcare.

Another internal audience would be the organization's *board of directors*. In most organizations the board of directors is charged with setting the direction of the organization and monitoring its progress. This body typically plays a critical role in the operation of the organization and should be considered an important customer by the staff of the organization.

There are other "secondary" audiences that should be considered as well. One of these is the *general public*. Most provider organizations and many other types of organizations in healthcare must maintain a positive public image. Not only is it important to create and sustain corporate goodwill, but it may be necessary to demonstrate at some point that the organization is a good community citizen and, in the case of not-for-profit organizations, that it deserves to retain its tax-exempt status.

Another audience for healthcare organizations is the *media*. The media requires cultivation in order to assure that the organization's story is told and told in the right manner. Indeed, long before hospitals and other healthcare organizations had formal marketing functions, they had public relations departments to deal with the media.

For many healthcare organizations, one or more branches of *government* represent audiences. Health facilities and health professions that are regulated by government agencies often maintain separate government relations offices. If the organization is not-for-profit, its tax-exempt status depends on maintaining good relationships with the appropriate government agencies. In areas where certificate-of-need requirements exist, healthcare organizations must maintain relationships with the appropriate agencies.

WHY HEALTHCARE AUDIENCES ARE DIFFERENT

Healthcare audiences differ from audiences in other industries in a variety of ways. To a great extent, health-related actions are non-discretionary. That is, they are often "ordered" by a health professional for the good of the patient. The patient could, of course, refuse the treatment, but that is not going to happen very often. There is virtually no other situation in any industry where a good or service is "prescribed" for the consumer and then pressure placed on the consumer to comply with the prescription.

Healthcare audiences are also distinguished from those in other industrial sectors by their insulation from the price of the products they consume. Because of the unusual financing arrangements characterizing healthcare and the lack of access to pricing information, healthcare consumers seldom know the price of the services they are consuming until after they have consumed them. In the typical case, in fact, the physician or clinician providing the service is also likely to not know the price of the services being provided. Since the end-user is seldom required to pay directly for the service—this is left up to third-party payers in the typical case—they may not even notice how much their care costs.

Healthcare audiences are hampered by a lack of knowledge on the cost of care and on other issues as well. Few consumers are knowledgeable concerning the operation of the healthcare system or have direct experience with many aspects of healthcare delivery. There is typically no basis for the evaluation of the quality of services provided by health facilities or practitioners, leaving the consumer with no means to make meaningful distinctions. Consumers must make judgments based on the provider's reputation or on superficial factors such as the appearance of the facilities, the available amenities, or the tastiness of the hospital's food. The consumer is left with no means for comparing services and the marketer with no real basis for differentiation.

Another factor setting healthcare audiences apart from other consumers is the personal nature of the services involved. While few healthcare encounters involve matters of life or death, virtually all of them involve an emotional component that is absent in other consumer transactions. Every diagnostic test is fraught with the possibility of a "positive" result, and every surgery, no matter how minor, carries the potential for complications. Today's well-informed consumers are aware of the level of medical errors characterizing hospital care and the amount of system-induced morbidity that occurs in healthcare settings. Even if individuals remain stoic with regard to their own care, they are likely to exhibit an emotional dimension when the care concerns a parent, a child or some other loved one. Whether this emotionally charged and personal aspect of the healthcare episode prevents the affected individual from seeking care, colors the choice of provider or therapy, or leads to additional symptoms, the choices made by the patient or other decision makers are likely to be affected. It is not unusual for emotions like fear, pride and vanity come into play. (Exhibit 5.1 presents differences between healthcare consumers and other types of consumers.)

WHY HEALTHCARE AUDIENCES ARE SIMILAR

While much has been made of the unique characteristics of health-care audiences, they are perhaps more similar to those in other industries than the above discussion would suggest. While some healthcare episodes involve emergency and/or life-threatening conditions, the overwhelming majority does not. Indeed, if the incredible volume of self-care episodes are factored into the equation, one might argue that what be considered a true medical episode is relatively rare.

It is clearly the case that a large proportion of the healthcare episodes that occur involves some discretion on the part of the end-user or those involved in the decision-making process and that the consumption of many types of services is "elective." For this reason, healthcare audiences can be considered to be similar to other audiences in many ways. For example, healthcare consumers are likely to distinguish between needs and wants when it comes to the consumption of services. Clearly, most healthcare consumers would consider angioplasty to correct a heart condition (a need), while laser eye surgery would be considered a want. The latter might be considered a discretionary expenditure while the former would be non-discretionary. Similarly, cardiac care would more than likely be considered a necessity, while for most consumers laser eye surgery would be considered a "luxury" purchase.

Healthcare consumers are like other consumers in that the level of demand for goods and services is elastic. Years ago the conventional wisdom was that the demand for health services was essentially inelastic. It was assumed that those who were sick consumed services and those who were well did not. Not only does this assumption reflect a dated notion of health and illness, but it does not account for the vast amount of discretionary transactions that occur in healthcare. We now realize that the demand for health services is extremely elastic and that the level of demand can be influenced by a wide range of factors—from the characteristics of the consumers themselves to the availability of services to patients' access to health insurance.

Further, we now realize that the demand for health services can be manipulated. Throughout this book, many cases will be cited in which consumers are made aware of a service that they previously did not know existed. Indeed, many consumers have been convinced that they had a condition that they did not know they suffered from. In the former case, emotionally disturbed individuals may be made aware of the availability of counseling services that they were unaware of. In the latter situation, parents may realize that their child has an attention deficit disorder or an individual may realize as a result of health communication that her "indigestion" is actually a gastric reflux disorder.

Exhibit 5.1

Healthcare Consumers vs. Other Consumers

Consumers of Health Services	*Consumers of Other Services*
Seldom determine their need for services	Usually determine their need for services
Seldom the ultimate decision maker	Usually the ultimate decision maker
Often subjective basis for decision	Usually objective basis for decision
Seldom has knowledge of the price	Always has knowledge of the price
Seldom makes decision based on price	Usually makes decision based on price
Cost mostly covered by a third party	Cost virtually never covered by a third party
Usually non-discretionary purchase	Usually discretionary purchase
Usually requires a professional referral	Almost never requires a professional referral
Limited choice among available options	No limit to choice among available options
Limited knowledge of service attributes	Significant knowledge of service attributes
Limited ability to judge quality of service	Usually able to judge quality of service
Limited ability to evaluate outcome	Able to evaluate outcome
Little recourse for unfavorable outcome	Ample recourse for unfavorable outcome
Seldom the ultimate target for marketing	Always the ultimate target for marketing
Not susceptible to standard marketing techniques	Susceptible to standard marketing techniques

Source: Thomas, Richard K. (2004). *Marketing Health Services*. Chicago: Health Administration Press.

SEGMENTING HEALTHCARE AUDIENCES

Any communication effort must be attuned to the needs and wants of different intended audiences. Given the diversity of the general public, trying to reach everyone with one message or strategy may result in an approach that does not effectively reach those most able or ready to respond.

Defining subgroups of a population according to common characteristics is called segmentation. Segmentation can help the communicator develop messages, materials, and activities that are relevant to the intended audience's current behavior and specific needs, preferences, beliefs, cultural attitudes, knowledge, and reading habits. It also helps to identify the best channels for reaching each group, because populations differ on factors such as access to information, the information sources they find reliable, and how they prefer to learn.

Not every subgroup within a population qualifies as a target market and there are certain rules of thumb that help marketers identify a meaningful market segment. A viable market segment should be *measurable* in that accurate and complete information on audience characteristics can be acquired in a cost-effective manner. It should be *accessible* in that it is possible to communicate effectively with the chosen segment using standard information dissemination methods. It should be *substantial* enough to be considered for separate marketing activity. And a segment should be *meaningful* in that it includes consumers who have attributes relevant to the aims of the communicator. In examining market segmentation as applied to healthcare, Berkowitz (1996) adds that a viable market segment should also evidence a desire for the product and have the ability to pay for it.

Audience segmentation can take a number of different forms and some of the more common are described below.

Demographic Segmentation. Audience segmentation on the basis of demographics is the best known of the approaches to identifying target markets. The links between demographic characteristics and health status, health-related attitudes, and health behavior have been well established. For this reason, demographic segmentation is always an early task in any communication initiative, and demographically distinct subgroups are typically defined relative to various goods and services.

Geographic Segmentation. An understanding of the spatial distribution of the target audience has become increasingly important as healthcare has become more consumer driven. One of the implications of this trend has been the increased emphasis on the appropriate location of health facilities. The market-driven approach to health services has demanded that healthcare organizations take their services to the population, and the major purchasers of health services are insisting on convenient locations for their enrollees. Knowledge of the manner in which the population is distributed within the service area and the linkage between geographic segmentation and other forms of segmentation is critical for the development of a marketing plan.

Psychographic Segmentation. For many types of goods and services an understanding of the psychographic or lifestyle characteristics of the target audience is essential. The lifestyle clusters that can be identified for a population often transcend (or at least complement) its demographic characteristics. Most importantly, psychographic traits can be linked to the attitudes, perceptions and expectations of the target audience, as well as to its propensity to purchase various services and products. While psychographic analysis in healthcare has lagged behind its use in other industries, health professionals are finding increasing number of applications for this approach and growing amounts of healthcare data are being incorporated into psychographic segmentation systems.

Usage Segmentation. A common form of segmentation long used by marketers is now being applied to healthcare. The market area population can be divided into categories based on the extent of use of a particular service. In the case of urgent care clinic usage, for example, the population can be divided into heavy users, moderate users, occasional users and non-users. This approach can be applied to a wide range of services, of course, but may have its most important applications when elective goods and services are under consideration. This information provides a basis for subsequent communication initiatives that can be tailored differently, for example, for existing loyal customers and non-customers. The willingness of individuals to respond to a communication initiative often reflects the extent to which they fall into the category of "adopters".

Payor Segmentation. A form of market segmentation unique to healthcare involves targeting audiences on the basis of their payor categories. The existence of insurance coverage and the type of coverage available are major considerations in the marketing of most health services. Further, health plans cover some services and not others, and this becomes an important consideration in marketing. For elective services that are paid for out of pocket, a targeted marketing approach is typically required. The payor mix of the target audience has now come to be one of the first considerations in consumer profiling.

Benefit Segmentation. Different people buy the same or similar products for different reasons. Benefit segmentation is based on the idea consumers can be grouped according to the principal benefit sought. The benefits that consumers consider when making a purchase decision related to a given good or service include such product attributes as quality, convenience, value, and ease of access.

A segmentation analysis may begin by comparing the characteristics of those who exhibit different behaviors. People who share similar characteristics may be very different in terms of health behavior. For example, consider two 55-year-old African-American women. They work together in the same department. They have the same amount of education and comparable household incomes. They live next door to each other, attend the same church, and often invite each other's family over for meals. They enjoy the same television shows, listen to the same radio stations, and often discuss articles that they both read in the paper. Neither has a family history of breast cancer, and both had children before age 30. Yet one woman goes for annual mammograms and the other has never had one. A demographic, physical, or cultural segmentation would group these women together, yet one is a member of the intended audience for a health communication initiative about mammography and the other is not (National Cancer Institute, 2003).

Differences have been clearly demonstrated in the case of lifestyles in market segments. Many populations that appear to be similar demographically may vary enough on lifestyle characteristics to require different approaches. This was discovered twenty years ago when it was still believed that all senior citizens were very much alike. It was found that differences in lifestyle characteristics among the elderly created a number of subgroups, all with somewhat different healthcare orientations despite their very similar demographic characteristics. (Psychographic segmentation is descussed in more detail below.).

PROFILING THE TARGET AUDIENCE

Once the intended audiences have been specified, additional information is likely to be required beyond that gathered during the initial research. The information collected depends on the objective of the health communication initiative. The approach also depends upon the amount of existing secondary research and the resources available to conduct primary research.

The target audience can be profiled along a number of different dimensions depending on the project being undertaken. The major categories of information that are likely to have implications for communication include demographic characteristics and lifestyle characteristics, along with attitudes, preferences and expectations. The key characteristics are presented below and discussed in more detail in Chapter 6.

Demographic Data

Demographic data serve as the foundation for most communication analyses. Not only are demographic data important for profiling the target audience, but they serve as the basis for the calculation of a number of statistics relevant to the planning analysis. While an understanding of the demographic composition of the target population is important in its own right, this information is also essential for identifying the prevalence of health conditions and determining utilization patterns within the community. These traits also provide insights into the approach to communication appropriate for various target audiences.

For our purposes, it is useful to categorize demographic variables into *biosocial* variables and *sociocultural* variables. Biosocial characteristics are clearly distinguished as demographic variables by their link to biological traits. The demographic variables included in this category are: *age, sex* and *race*. (*Ethnicity* is sometimes included because of its close relationship to race.)

Age is probably the best single predictor of a number of health-related variables. Age is related not only to levels of service utilization but to the type of services utilized and the circumstances under which they are received.

The *sex* of the consumer is another factor influencing utilization rates in U.S. society. Females are more active than males in terms of health behavior and are heavier users of the healthcare system. They tend to visit physicians more often, take more prescription drugs, and, in general, use other facilities and personnel more often.

The *population pyramid* is a useful way of simultaneously depicting the age and sex structure of a population graphically. A population pyramid involves a presentation of the age-sex distribution of a population by means of a bar graph where each bar represents one age-sex group. Female age cohorts comprise one side of each bar and males the other and the ages are typically presented in five- or ten-year intervals. The "shape" of the pyramid discloses a great deal of information about the population in question and this information can be converted into estimates of the demand for health services.

Racial and ethnic characteristics influence the demand for health services, and, as a result of recent trends, this aspect of population composition is becoming increasingly important for health communicators. Detailed information on the racial and ethnic characteristics of the population should be compiled, including qualitative data on attitudes and preferences. While differences in utilization may be traced to differences in the types of health problems experienced by these populations, many of the distinctions reflect variations in lifestyle patterns and cultural preferences.

Sociocultural traits are important in profiling the population because of their correlation with health status and health behavior. Further, the sociocultural context of targeted individuals is typically a determinant of their communication styles. The sociocultural variables discussed below include: marital status and related attributes, education, income, occupation/industry, and other sociocultural factors. Additional information on insurance coverage, psychographic categories, and consumer attitudes is included. (See Box 5.1 for a discussion of culturally competent communication.)

Box 5.1

Developing Culturally Sensitive Communications

Culture encompasses the values, norms, symbols, ways of living, traditions, history, and institutions shared by a group of people. Cultural traits affect the ways in which people perceive and respond to health messages and materials, and are intertwined with health behaviors. Often, an individual is influenced by more than one culture; for example, teenagers are influenced by their individual family cultures as well as the norms, values, and symbols that comprise teen culture in their community.

To develop an effective health communication initiative, it is important to understand key aspects of the cultures or subcultures influencing the intended audience and build that understanding into the communication strategy. Messages must take into account cultural norms in terms of what is asked (e.g., don't ask people to make a behavior change that would violate cultural norms), what benefit is promised in exchange (in some cultures, community is most important; in others, individual benefit is), and what image is portrayed. The symbols, metaphors, visuals (including clothing, jewelry, and hairstyles), types of actors, language, and music used in materials all carry meaning.

While it is important to acknowledge and understand the cultures within an intended audience, developing separate messages and materials for each cultural group is not always necessary or even advisable. Careful intended audience research can help the program identify messages and images that resonate across groups—or identify situations in which different messages or images are likely to work best.

According to a Center for Substance Abuse Prevention *Technical Assistance Bulletin*, culturally sensitive communications:

- Acknowledge culture as a predominant force in shaping behaviors, values, and institutions
- Are based on concepts and materials developed for and with the involvement of the intended audience.
- Refer to cultural groups using terms that members of the group prefer

Box 5.1 (Continued).

- Use the language of the intended audience, carefully developed and tested with the involvement of the audience
- Take into consideration the predominant attitudes toward the healthcare system and health professionals.

Marital status, household structure and, to a degree, *living arrangements* are all of interest to health communicators. Marital status refers to one's current legal status with regard to marriage. Household structure refers to involvement in the physical household–i.e., where one actually lives. Living arrangements refer to the relationship between those sharing a household–i.e., roommates, married with children, unmarried relatives. Marital status and household structure may have implications for the types of health problems that exist and the patterns of health services utilization.

Education is an extremely important factor to consider for communication purposes. This information is often important for the development of services that are compatible with the level of sophistication of the target audience. Certainly from a social marketing perspective, the level of education needs to be taken into consideration.

Income and related attributes, such as poverty status, are critical for communication planning. Income, measured in terms of annual household income or per capita income, is an important predictor of both the level of morbidity within the community and likely patterns of health services utilization. The overall level of community affluence will influence both the healthcare "wants" of the population and the level of resources available.

Occupation and *industry* are important variables in profiling a target audience. Not only do individuals in different occupations and industries have differing consumer behavior habits, but the occupational or industrial mix of an area is an excellent indicator of the mix of healthcare goods and services required by the target population. Distinctive patterns of healthy and unhealthy behavior have been correlated with different occupations and industries.

There are other sociocultural characteristics that might be important in different communities. Religion is a characteristic of the population that is difficult to measure and has, in fact, played a limited role in communication planning. However, there are occasions when knowledge of a community's religious preferences may be appropriate for communication planning, especially if there are strong ties to church-affiliated health facilities in the community under study. The language spoken by the community population or sub-populations may also be a factor influencing healthcare communication and the efficient delivery of services.

Other Segmentation Considerations

As noted earlier, has become increasingly common to profile consumers in terms of their *psychographic characteristics* and assign them to lifestyle clusters. Psychographics refers to the values, attitudes and lifestyles that characterize a defined population segment. Lifestyle segmentation systems have been developed by a variety of vendors but they have only recently come into use in healthcare. The approach involves dividing the population into a large number of segments (usually 50–60) that can then be profiled in terms of various characteristics including health status and health behavior. Psychographic factors are particularly important in examining attitudes towards one's health and the likelihood of involvement in healthy or unhealthy behaviors. Methods of communicating are typically a reflection of one's lifestyle characteristics.

Psychographic analysis can help determine the likely health priorities and behaviors of a population subgroup. This is important because groups that are similar demographically may be different in terms of their lifestyle-influenced health behavior. For example, one category of elderly healthcare consumers may prefer general practitioners for their primary care needs, while another category prefers physicians trained in internal medicine. Knowledge of the psychographic clusters characterizing a target audience provides a useful guide for the development of health communication initiatives.

The *attitudes* characterizing the target audience is another dimension that must be considered. "Attitudes" may encompass perceptions, preferences and expectations. The attitudes displayed by consumers will have important implications for communication. The impact of health education programs and prevention initiatives are likely to be greatly influenced by consumer attitudes.

The community's attitudes, for example, may reflect a pro-physician or pro-hospital stance. In other cases there may be strong positive or negative perceptions (whether based on fact or not) with regard to various institutions or providers. There may be preferences for certain types of practitioners or methods of treatment over others. Some target audiences may be very traditional in their attitudes toward healthcare, while others may be quick to embrace alternative treatment modalities.

Another important consideration is the *cultural preferences* of the target population. These cultural preferences (often reflected in lifestyles) may not be directly related to health behavior although many are. Social group preferences for marital status or family size may affect the health status of the population. More directly, dietary habits, exercise patterns, and patterns of unhealthy behavior (e.g., smoking and alcohol use) affect the health status of the population and ultimately the demand for health services. To the extent that healthy or unhealthy behavior is encouraged by the individual's cultural context, this is an important consideration for health communicators.

References

National Cancer Institute. (2003). *Making health communication work*. Washington: US Government Printing Office.

Additional Resources

Center for Substance Abuse Prevention. (1994). *Following specific guidelines will help you assess cultural competence in program design, application, and management* Technical Assistance Bulletin, Washington, DC: US Government Printing Office.

Glanz, K., Lewis, F. M., & Rimer, B. K. (Eds.). (1997). *Health behavior and health education: Theory, research, and practice* (2nd ed.). San Francisco: Jossey-Bass.

Glanz, K., & Rimer, B. K. (1995). *Theory at a glance: A guide for health promotion practice*. NIH Publication No. 97-3896. Bethesda, MD: National Cancer Institute.

Goldberg, M. E., Fishbein, M. F., & Middlestadt, S. E. (Eds.). (1997). *Social marketing: Theoretical and practical perspectives*. Mahwah, NJ: Erlbaum.

Maibach, E., & Parrott, R. L. (Eds.). (1995). *Designing health messages: Approaches from communication theory and public health practice*. Thousand Oaks, CA: Sage.

National Cancer Institute. (1994). *Clear and simple: Developing effective print materials for low-literate readers* (NIH Publication No. 95-3594). Bethesda, MD.

Palmgreen, P., et al. (1995). Reaching at-risk populations in a mass media drug abuse prevention campaign: Sensation seeking as a targeting variable. *Drugs and Society*, 8(3), 29–45.

Rimer, B. K., & Glassman, B. (1998). Tailoring communications for primary care settings. *Methods of Information in Medicine*, 37(3), 171–177.

Selden, C. R., Zorn, M., Ratzan, S., & Parker, R. M. (2000). *Health literacy, January 1990 through October 1999*. Bethesda, MD: National Library of Medicine.

Siegel, M., & Doner, L. (1998). *Marketing public health: Strategies to promote social change*. Gaithersburg, MD: Aspen.

Chapter 6

Understanding Health Behavior

Health communication is often utilized to influence health behavior. Chapter 6 reviews the various forms of health behavior and the factors that influence this behavior. Relevant theories formulated to explain health behavior are presented and their relevance to health communication discussed.

MODELS OF HEALTH BEHAVIOR

Numerous attempts have been made to develop explanatory frameworks for understanding health behavior. Different models have been developed geared to the individual, the group and the community (National Cancer Institute, 2003). Although there is no generally accepted model, the most important ones are described below.

Individual Level

One set of models of health behavior focuses on the individual level and considers how individuals make decisions with regard to health behavior. Effective communication under these types of models requires an in-depth understanding of individual traits and attributes.

Behavioral Intentions

Studies of behavioral intentions suggest that the likelihood of intended audiences' adopting a desired behavior can be predicted by assessing (and subsequently trying to change or influence) their attitudes toward and perceptions of benefits of the behavior. Research by Fishbein and Ajzen (1975) supports the idea that individuals and society's perceived attitudes are an important predecessor to action. Therefore, an important step toward influencing behavior is a preliminary assessment of intended audience attitudes, with subsequent tracking necessary to identify any attitudinal changes.

Stages of Change

The basic premise of the stages-of-change construct is that behavior change is a process and not an event. Further, individuals are considered to be at varying levels of motivation or readiness to change. The extent to which people are responsive to change will depend on their stage at that point in time.

Knowing an individual's current stage allows communicators to set realistic program goals. It is possible to tailor messages, strategies, and programs to the appropriate stage. Five distinct stages have been identified in the stages-of-change construct:

1. Precontemplation
2. Contemplation
3. Decision/determination
4. Action
5. Maintenance

It is important to note that this is a circular, not a linear, model. Individuals can enter or exit at any point and recycle back through the model.

Health Belief Model

The health belief model (HBM) was originally designed to explain why people did not participate in programs to prevent or detect diseases. The core components of the HBM include:

- Perceived susceptibility—the subjective perception of risk of developing a particular health condition
- Perceived severity—feelings about the seriousness of the consequences of developing a specific health problem
- Perceived benefits—beliefs about the effectiveness of various actions that might reduce susceptibility and severity
- Perceived barriers—potential negative aspects of taking specific actions
- Cues to action—bodily or environmental events that trigger action

More recently, the HBM has been amended to include the notion of self-efficacy as another predictor of health behaviors, especially more complex ones in which lifestyle changes must be maintained over time. A wide variety of demographic, social, psychological, and structural variables may also impact people's perceptions and, indirectly, their health-related behaviors. Some of the more important variables include educational attainment, age, gender, socioeconomic status, and prior knowledge.

Consumer Information Processing Model

The consumer information processing (CIP) model was not developed specifically to study health-related behavior, nor to be applied in a health communication context, but it has many useful applications in the health arena. Information is a common tool for health education and is often an essential foundation for health decisions. The conveyance of information can increase or decrease people's anxiety, depending on their information preferences and the amount and kind of information they are given.

Illness and its treatments can interfere with information processing. By understanding the key concepts and processes of CIP, health educators can examine why people use or fail to use health information and subsequently design more effective communication strategies. CIP theory reflects a combination of rational and motivational ideas. The use of information is an intellectual process; however, motivation drives the search for information and how much attention people pay to it.

The central assumptions of CIP are that 1) individuals are limited in how much information they can process, and 2) to increase the usability of information, healthcare consumers combine bits of information into "chunks" and create decision rules to make choices faster and more easily. According to basic CIP concepts, before people will use health information, it must be: 1) available; 2) seen as useful and new; and, 3) processable.

Interpersonal Level

Another type of model posits that behavior is a function of the influence of interpersonal relationships in which the individual is involved. These relationships provide clues—if not outright direction—for behavior. Effective communication must take into consideration the different forces that are generated through interpersonal transactions as demonstrated by the one example offered below.

Social Cognitive Theory

Social cognitive theory (SCT) explains behavior in terms of triadic reciprocality ("reciprocal determinism") in which behavior, cognitive and other interpersonal factors, and environmental events all operate as inter-acting determinants of one another. SCT describes behavior as dynamically determined and fluid, influenced by both personal factors and the environment. Changes in any of these three factors are hypothesized to engender changes in the others.

SCT views the environment as not just a variable that reinforces or punishes behaviors, but one that also provides a milieu in which an individual can watch the actions of others and learn the consequences of those behaviors. Processes governing observational learning include:

- *Attention*—gaining and maintaining attention
- *Retention*—being remembered
- *Reproduction*—reproducing the observed behavior
- *Motivation*—being stimulated to produce the behavior

Organization/Community/Societal Level

A third type of model operates at the more macro levels of organization, community and society. Communication activities at these levels may be geared to influencing organizational change, modifying the environment of the community, or influencing public policy. Given this, communication efforts under this model are likely to take a variety of forms and be particularly complex.

Organizational Change Theory

Organizations represent complex social systems composed of many components. Organizational change can best be promoted by working at multiple levels within the organization. Understanding organizational change is important for establishing policies and environments that support healthy practices and create the capacity to solve new problems. While there are many theories of organization behavior, two are especially of interest to us here: stage theory and organizational development (OD) theory.

Stage theory is based on the idea that organizations pass through a series of steps or stages as they change. Strategies to promote change can be matched to various points in the process of change. An abbreviated version of stage theory involves four stages:

- Problem definition (awareness)
- Initiation of action (adoption)
- Implementation
- Institutionalization

OD theory grew out of the recognition that organizational structures and processes influence worker behavior and motivation. OD theory concerns the identification of problems that impede an organization's functioning, rather than the introduction of a specific type of change. A typical OD strategy involves process consultation, in which an outside specialist helps identify problems and facilitates the planning of change strategies (including communication approaches).

Stage theory and OD theory have the greatest potential to produce health-enhancing change in organizations when they are combined. That is, OD strategies can be used at various stages as they are warranted. Simultaneously, the stages signal the need to involve organization members and decision-makers at various points in the process.

Community Organization Theory

Community organization theory has its origin in theories of social networks and support. It emphasizes active participation in developing communities that can better evaluate and solve health and social problems. Community organization is the process by which community groups identify common problems, mobilize resources, and develop and implement strategies for reaching specified goals. It has its roots in several theoretical perspectives: the ecological perspective, social systems perspective, social networks, and social support. It is also consistent with social learning theory (SLT) and can be successfully used along with SLT-based strategies. Some approaches to community change include:

- *Locality development* (also called community development) uses a broad cross-section of people in the community to identify and solve its own problems. It stresses consensus development, capacity building, and a strong task orientation; outside practitioners help to coordinate and enable the community to successfully address its concerns.
- *Social planning* uses tasks and goals, and addresses substantive problem solving, with expert practitioners providing technical assistance to benefit community members.
- *Social action* aims to increase the problem-solving ability of the community and to achieve concrete changes to redress social injustice that is identified by a disadvantaged or oppressed group.

Although community organization theory does not use a single unified model, several key concepts are central to the various approaches. The process of empowerment is intended to stimulate problem solving and activate community members. Community competence is an approximate community-level equivalent of self-efficacy plus behavioral capability, which involves the confidence and skills to solve problems effectively. Participation and relevance involve citizen activation and a collective sense of readiness for change. Issue selection concerns identifying "winnable battles" as a focus for action, and critical consciousness stresses the active search for root causes of problems. Of course, health communication is a basic component of each of these dimensions of social intervention.

Diffusion of Innovations Theory

Diffusion of innovations theory addresses how new ideas, products, and social practices spread within a society or from one society to another. The challenge of diffusion requires approaches that differ from those focused solely on individuals or small groups. This approach requires attention to the innovation (a new idea, product, practice, or technology) as well as to communication channels and social systems (networks with members, norms, and social structures).

A focus on the characteristics of innovations can improve the chances that they will be adopted and hence diffused. It also has implications for the positioning of an innovation to maximize its appeal. Some of the most important characteristics of innovations are their:

- *Relative advantage*—is it better than what was there before?
- *Compatibility*—fit with intended audience
- *Complexity*—ease of use
- *Trialability*—can it be tried out first?
- *Observability*—visibility of results

Communication channels are another important component of diffusion of innovations theory. Diffusion theories view communication as a two-way process rather than one of merely "persuading" an intended audience to take action. The two-step flow of communication—in which opinion leaders mediate the impact of mass media—emphasizes the value of social networks (or interpersonal channels) over and above mass media for adoption decisions.

HEALTH BEHAVIOR PATTERNS

The factors that determine the perceptions, attitudes and preferences of healthcare consumers—and by extension their behavior—include demographic characteristics, lifestyle characteristics, and insurance characteristics, as well as the health conditions that they face. The demographic factors that affect health behavior patterns are summarized in the sections that follow.

   Age is considered by many to be the single best predictor of the utilization of health services, the amount and type of services used, and the circumstances under which they are received. Although it has become a truism in U.S. society that the consumption of health services increases with age, this primarily reflects the heavy weight accorded to hospital care. In terms of emergency room utilization (for true emergencies), teens and those in their early twenties along with the elderly account for a disproportionate share due to injuries and accidents.

   Age differences exist in the utilization of physician services, although they are not as dramatic as those for hospital and nursing home services. With the exception of the youngest age cohorts, there is a direct relationship between age and number of physician office visits. A significant difference exists in the utilization of specialists and the age of the patient. With increases in age, the utilization rate for primary care physicians decreases and that for specialists increases.

   The relationship between nursing home utilization and age is predictable. Few nursing home residents are under 65. However, within the nursing home population itself, there are significant differences in age distribution. A similar pattern exists with regard to the use of hospice services (National Center for Health Statistics 2002, tables 88 and 89).

   Age differences are also found in the use of other types of facilities. Among the older population, there is a preference for inpatient rather than outpatient care. The ingrained notion of better care and a more secure environment among older age cohorts tends to favor hospitalization. On the other hand, preferences for outpatient settings among the younger age cohorts have emerged. The primary users of freestanding urgent care clinics, for example, are in the 25 to 40 age group. The under-45 population is also more likely to utilize other outpatient settings, such as freestanding diagnostic centers or surgicenters. These differences are partly a reflection of age-generated differences in perceptions. But they also reflect the fact that younger age cohorts are more likely to be enrolled in some alternative delivery system that mandates outpatient care and to have physicians with more "contemporary" practice patterns than those of the older age groups.

   Since age is considered one of the most important correlates of health services utilization, the implications of age for health communication are highly significant. Important differences in the sources of information can be identified for different age groups, and variations in the message, channel and timing can all be expected for various age groups. For example, youth are likely to gain much of their health-related information from the Internet, while seniors are more likely to look to some authority figure such as a physician for health-related information.

   The *sexual makeup* of a population is also likely to influence its health behavior. In U.S. society, females are more proactive than men with regard to healthcare and are consequently much heavier users of the healthcare system. They tend to visit physicians more often, take more prescription drugs, and use other facilities and personnel in general more often. Obviously women will consume all services of OB/GYNs, but they are also over-represented in general practice settings due to their higher prevalence of chronic conditions. Driven by the use of obstetrical services, hospital utilization was significantly greater for females than males in 2000 (National Center for Health Statistics, 2002, table 90).

Females comprise the majority of nursing home admissions, and the nation's nursing home population is nearly 75 percent female. For the 85-and-over cohort, the female proportion is over 80 percent (National Center for Health Statistics 2002, table 97). The higher mortality rate for males, coupled with the lower survival rate for males who do become ill, means that there are more female candidates for nursing home admission. Further, males surviving into the older age cohorts are more likely to have a wife to care for them. Women also account for nearly two-thirds of home health patients.

Those involved in communication in any field realize that men and women acquire, process and interpret information in different ways. Both males and females raise important considerations for communicators but for different reasons. In the U.S. communicating health-related information to men is a challenge, resulting in a large hard-to-reach population. Women, while more easily reached through communication, require messages that reflect their particular needs and recognize the fact that they control the majority of healthcare decisions made within the population.

A correlation has been found between *racial and ethnic characteristics* and the utilization of certain types of health services. The most clear-cut differences have been identified between the sickness behavior of African Americans and whites. Certain Asian populations and ethnic groups also display somewhat distinctive utilization patterns. To a limited extent, differences in utilization may be traced to differences in the types of health problems experienced. However, many of the differences in the use of healthcare resources reflect variations in lifestyle patterns and cultural preferences.

The hospital admission rate for whites tends to be around 20 percent lower than that for African Americans, despite the older age structure of the white population. Discharge rates for Asian-Americans and Hispanics are much lower than those for whites, while those for American Indians are in between the white and black rates (National Center for Health Statistics, 2002, table 90).

Whites are over-represented among the nursing home population. African Americans and other racial and ethnic groups tend to be under-represented, although Hispanics increasingly report a pattern similar to that of non-Hispanic whites. This under-representation among African Americans is particularly telling in view of the heavy burden of chronic disease and disability affecting that population.

Whites are also over-represented among the patients of specialists. While African Americans are over-represented among the patients of obstetricians (primary care), they are under-represented among the clients of ophthalmologists and orthopedic surgeons (specialty care).

Blacks are significantly more likely to utilize emergency room services than are whites. The rate of emergency room use for Hispanics is similar to that for whites, while American Indians have the highest emergency room use rates of any racial group. Asian-Americans are the least likely to use emergency room services of any group (National Center for Health Statistics, 2002, table 79).

Some ethnic group members (Hispanics, for example) utilize alternative types of care in the form of "traditional" healers. Thus, their physician utilization rate does not provide a full picture of their healthcare utilization. In fact, recent research into the use of alternative therapies by Americans suggests that the whole notion of the utilization of clinic services needs to be reviewed (Eisenberg and Kessler, 1993).

The racial and ethnic profile of the U.S. population is highly complex and is becoming even more so. This is an area in which vast differences are likely to be found with regard to knowledge, attitudes and perceptions. These differences are exacerbated by cultural differences unrelated to healthcare that may influence their interaction with the healthcare system. Overlay on this the language barriers that are likely to exist, and the health communicator faces some significant challenges. However, these are challenges that must be addressed given the growing influence of race and ethnicity on health behavior.

Marital status is a surprisingly effective predictor of the utilization of health services. Marital status is related not only to levels of service utilization but to the type of services utilized and the circumstances under which they are received. (The categories of marital status for the discussion below are never married, married, divorced, and widowed.)

In general, the married require fewer services because they are healthier. Yet, they utilize more of certain types of services because they are more aware of the need for preventive care, are more likely to have insurance, and, it is argued, have a "significant other" to encourage them to use the healthcare system.

The age-adjusted rate of hospitalization for married individuals is relatively low. Admission rates for the never married also tend to be relatively low, while those for the widowed and divorced are high by comparison. If rates of admission for various conditions are considered, the variation among marital statuses is even more pronounced.

Some differences related to marital status do exist in the utilization of physician services, although they are not as dramatic as those for hospital and nursing home services. Federal surveys have found that married women "see" a doctor (i.e., via visit or telephone) an average of seven times a year. The rate of contact for divorced and widowed women is slightly higher. The rate of physician contact for males is lower than that for females in every marital status category, although little difference exists from one marital status to another for men. Some differences exist in the utilization of specialists by the marital status of the patient, but these are not great.

The relationship between nursing home utilization and marital status is one of the most clear-cut to be discussed in this section. Few nursing home residents are married. The bulk of nursing home residents are widowed, although there are small numbers who are divorced or never married. Married individuals requiring nursing care are often maintained in the home and cared for by a spouse.

The importance of marital status and household structure for health communication is often neglected. Given the importance of the household context for the transmission of information on healthcare and any other topic for that matter, an understanding of the marital status and household characteristics of any population is critical. Family is an important source of health-related information, and the messages, channels, and timing are likely to vary widely depending on whether on is addressing population that includes couples only, couples with children, single parents, and so forth.

Income is probably one of the better predictors of the utilization of health services. Income is related not only to levels of service utilization but to the types of services utilized and the circumstances under which they are received. Hospitalization rates tend to decrease directly with income and, in fact, greater discrepancies exist among the various income groups than for any of the other social variables examined. The rate of hospitalization for the lowest income group in the U.S. is the highest of any income group, reflecting the higher incidence of health problems (National Center for Health Statistics, 2002, table 90).

Lower income groups are heavier users of hospital emergency room care, especially for non-emergency conditions. On the other hand, lower-income populations are less likely to utilize freestanding emergency clinics or urgent care clinics. This is presumably due to a lack of knowledge of their availability (they are often located in suburban areas) and the fact that payment is typically demanded when care is rendered.

Historically, the number of annual physician visits per capita increased as income increases. The lowest income groups tended to be infrequent users of physician services and, in the past, this reflected a lack of family physicians and the use of alternative sources of care such as public health clinics. This situation has changed since the 1960s due to the availability of government-sponsored insurance programs and programs that subsidize physician services in underserved communities. However, the lower income groups continue to be under-represented among the patients of private-practice physicians and over-represented among emergency department users (National Center for Health Statistics, 2002, table 79).

As income increases, the utilization rate of primary care physicians decreases and that of specialists increases (National Center for Health Statistics, 2002, table 85). There is also a direct and inverse relationship between income and dental care utilization. The more affluent see dental care as a preventive service, while the less affluent see it as an expensive service to be used only in emergencies.

Given the role that income plays in influencing health behavior in the U.S., the characteristics of various income groups should be well known to the health communicator. Some of the greatest differences in health behavior have been observed between the affluent and the poverty populations. The economic circumstances of various subgroups in society play a major role in establishing their attitudes, preferences, and expectations vis-à-vis healthcare.

The relationship between *education* and the use of health services resembles that for income, and educational level is probably one of the better predictors of the utilization of health services. Education is related not only to levels of service utilization but to the types of services utilized and the circumstances under which they are received.

The rate of hospitalization for the least educated segments of the U.S. population is very low, despite the fact that the incidence of health problems is greater for the poorly educated than for any other group. The better educated, although less affected by health problems, have much higher rates of hospitalization. This is thought to be a function of their greater appreciation of the benefits of healthcare and more insurance coverage on the part of the better educated.

Physician utilization is considerably higher for the best educated than for the least. In general, the number of annual physician visits per capita increases with education. The lowest educational groups record the lowest rates of physician visits. As education increases, the utilization rate for primary care physicians decreases and that of specialists increases. This partly reflects the prestige dimension of medical specialists and the knowledge required to select a specialist. The presumed greater expertise of specialists makes them appealing to the well educated.

Less-educated groups are heavier users of hospital emergency room care, especially for non-emergency conditions. On the other hand, better-educated populations are more likely to utilize urgent care centers. The better educated are also more likely to utilize other outpatient settings, such as freestanding diagnostic centers or ambulatory surgery centers.

Some would argue that the educational level (or perhaps more specifically the literacy level) of the target population is the major consideration when it comes to health communication. Indeed, much of the research that has taken place related to health communication has focused on the implications of low literacy levels for an understanding of health conditions and subsequent health behavior.

Occupational status is related not only to levels of service utilization but to the types of services utilized and the circumstances under which they are received. In general, those in higher occupational categories require less services because they are healthier. Yet, they utilize more of certain types of services because they are more aware of the need for preventive care and tend to have better insurance coverage.

Higher status occupational groups have somewhat higher admission rates. The pattern identified for the various occupational statuses for patient days is comparable to that for admissions. The lower-status occupational categories make up for any differences in admissions by recording more patient days.

Some differences are found in the use of other types of facilities on the basis of occupational status. Income and educational levels no doubt play a role here, and the type of insurance coverage available (which is primarily a function of employment status) is important in the type of service utilized. Some differences related to occupational status do exist in the utilization of physician services.

The occupational characteristics of those in a targeted population have important implications for health communication. Along with income and educational levels, the type of occupation, the industry employed in, and the status of the occupation can affect the perceptions, attitudes, and expectations of those in different occupational circumstances and these will ultimately affect health behavior.

CONSUMER BEHAVIOR

"Consumer behavior" refers to the patterns of consumption of goods and services that characterize healthcare consumers, along with the factors that contribute to this behavior and processes that communication often focuses on. In healthcare the behavior of the end-user is only one type of behavior to be considered—and a recent one to come to the attention of health professionals at that. Since health communication must be responsive to consumer characteristics, an appreciation of the behavioral dimension of any target population is essential. It is ultimately this behavior that the health communicator seeks to influence.

Decisions with regard to the use of health services are influenced by many factors, a lot of which do not play a role in other consumption decisions. These decisions are likely to involve an emotional component, and healthcare consumers may be facing life-threatening situations that affect them or their loved ones. The fact that many consumers cannot bring themselves to even say the word "cancer" supports this view. Emotions like fear, pride and vanity come into play. For example, who would have thought 20 years ago that men would overtake women in the use of cosmetic surgery?

Despite the differences between healthcare consumers and other consumers, the decision criteria for healthcare consumers can be classified in the same manner as those in other industries. The types of factors that influence purchase decisions include technical, economic, social and personal criteria. Technical criteria include quality of care, clinical outcomes, environment, and the amenities that influence the decisions of healthcare consumers. Economic factors, perhaps the least relevant in healthcare, include the price of goods and services, the mechanism for payment (e.g., insurance), and the perceived value of the service rendered. Social criteria include such factors as the status associated with the professional, facility or procedure performed, the influence of the social group, and other factors related to the social environment. Personal criteria include factors related to the emotional aspects of the service, self-image issues, and even moral and ethical considerations.

It is traditional to think in terms of a hierarchy of needs in setting the context for the analysis of consumer decision making. Most refer to Maslow's theory of motivation in addressing this issue (Maslow, 1970). Maslow contended that the first order of need for human beings involved physiological needs for food, water, air, shelter, sex, etc. Once these basic needs are met, society members can begin to think in terms of their safety and security needs. These would include freedom from various threats and the establishment of security, order, and predictability in their lives. It is at this stage that "health" begins to emerge as à value in its own right.

With this foundation, society members can begin to think in terms of social or companionship needs, the next level in the hierarchy. These include friendship, affection, and a sense of belonging. To these needs would eventually be added esteem or ego needs. These would include the need for self-respect along with self-confidence, competence, achievement, independence, and prestige. Finally, at the top of the needs hierarchy, individuals would have a felt need for self-actualization. This includes the fulfillment of personal potential through education, career development, and general personal fulfillment. Few societies in the history of the world, of course, have achieved this level of need fulfillment for any significant portion of their population.

This model has important implications for health communication. First, the level of the hierarchy at which an individual or a population functions says a lot about the healthcare needs it faces. At the lower levels of the model, survival needs dominate the healthcare arena. Society members face threats from pathological agents and from a hostile environment. At the higher levels of the model, the threats common at the lowest levels have been moderated and, rather than attempting to preserve life and limb, society members can focus on health maintenance and enhancement. Their needs shift from life-saving procedures and public health considerations to self-actualization needs such as weight control, fitness programs, and cosmetic surgery.

From a health communication perspective, individuals who are at the survival level are only likely to be responsive to information that addresses their immediate needs. They are not going to respond to promotions for services that enhance their quality of life or require out-of-pocket expenditures. (This helps explain the difficulty involved in convincing financially precarious individuals that they ought to invest in healthy lifestyles.) As individuals progress up the hierarchy, they are more open to discretionary services and appreciate the importance of maintaining and enhancing their health status. In effect, they are open to a different form of communication.

Ultimately, the method for reaching individuals at different levels in the needs hierarchy, and the message that is appropriate will reflect one's position in this model. Health professionals are faced with the challenge of matching the product, medium and message to the status of the target audience vis-à-vis the needs hierarchy.

CONSUMER DECISION MAKING

In virtually every other industry, the end-user is responsible for the purchase decision, and it is the decision maker who actually consumes the good or service. This is often not the case in healthcare where the end-user of the service (e.g., the patient) often does not make the decision to purchase the service. Thus, a physician is likely to determine the what, where, when and how much of the service that is to be provided. Alternatively, the decision maker may be a health plan representative, an employer, or a family member, and not the party who eventually consumes the service. Health professionals are faced with the challenge of determining the manner in which to communicate under these circumstances.

Another unique characteristic of healthcare that has implications for health communication is the fact that the end-user of a service may not be the ultimate target of the communication initiative. In fact, health professionals have identified a number of other categories of target audiences that may be more important than the end-user. For example, various categories of *influencers* have been identified. These could be family members, counselors, or other health professionals that encourage consumers to use a particular good or service. The role of various *gatekeepers* might also be considered. These could include primary care physicians, insurance plan personnel, discharge planners, and others who have responsibility for channeling consumers into certain services. Any or all of these could be targets for communication.

Another category involves the *decision makers* who make choices for the consumer. These could be family members, primary care physicians, or caregivers who act on behalf of consumers for various reasons. Finally, there is a category of *buyers* of healthcare services that includes employers, business coalitions, and other groups that might indirectly control the behavior of consumers by determining which services they can and cannot utilize. (The role health communication plays in the patient "career" is discussed in Box 6.1.)

One of the most important findings from recent research relates to the importance of women in the healthcare decision-making process. It has already been established that women utilize a disproportionate share of healthcare resources. By virtue of being inordinately heavy users of health services for themselves, women effectively make the majority of purchase decisions on the consumer side. Further, women generally make most of the decisions for their children and often their husbands as well. They are also likely to be involved as healthcare decision makers for their parents or other dependent family members. While women consume at least half of the personal health services in the U.S., they could conceivably account for 80 percent or more of the decisions to purchase goods or use services.

A basic understanding of the process that consumers go through in the purchase decision-making process is important for communication planning purposes (Berkowitz and Hillestad, 1991). The steps listed below in the decision-making process represent an amalgam of various approaches to this process overlaid with a healthcare perspective. The steps in the process include:

Problem Recognition. The first step in the purchase decision process occurs when the consumer recognizes a problem or need. The task for the communicator is to identify the circumstances and/or stimuli that trigger a particular need and use this knowledge to develop communication strategies that trigger consumer interest.

Information Search. At this stage of the decision process the consumer is aroused to search for more information. The consumer may evidence heightened attention to the condition or initiate an active information

Box 6.1

The Role of Communication in the Patient "Career"

The patient "career" can be viewed as a linear phenomenon in which an individual proceeds through a variety of stages. If the assumption is made that individuals are naturally in a state of "health," a scenario can be developed whereby prevention, screening, and routine self-care represent the initial stage. With the onset of symptoms, the individual makes a transition to the point of diagnosis and treatment at an outpatient facility. It is at this point that the symptomatic individual is "officially" defined as a patient and enters the formal care system. This may involve a variety of settings and practitioners for addressing the identified health problem.

Assuming the patient survives the illness episode, he or she may move out of the patient care model back into the community as a "well" person. Alternatively, the patient may require follow-up care or chronic disease management (e.g., by a home care agency), temporary institutionalized care (e.g., a subacute facility), long-term nursing care (e.g., a nursing home), or rehabilitative services of some type (e.g., physical or occupational therapy). These post-patient services extend the model horizontally. This patient "career" could actually be thought of as involving three stages: pre-patient, patient, and post-patient.

The characteristics of health communication vary depending on the stage of the career in terms of sources, contexts, channels, messages and timing. Early on in the process, the symptomatic individual, even prior to disclosing the symptoms to anyone, seeks out information from various sources. This may involve picking up literature at a healthcare facility, a social service office, or a health fair, or researching the symptoms at the library. Increasingly, healthcare consumers are accessing the Internet at the first appearance of symptoms.

Whether or not these sources of information adequately answer the questions, the symptomatic individual then typically turns to informal sources of information related to his or her condition. This means turning to family members, friends, and associates for information. Indeed, these informal sources of health information remain even today as mainstays for those seeking knowledge about a health condition. Individuals place considerable confidence in this form of communication, coming as it is from people that are trusted and who can be expected to have the best interests of the affected individual at heart. Personal forms of communication complement the impersonal sources of data previously accessed.

Box 6.1 (Continued).

As the patient career progresses, increasingly formal sources of input are sought, and the communication process takes a different form. In addition, information on the healthcare system is now required to supplement information on the health condition. Information seeking here may involve communication with a professional known to the affected individual or an accessible health professional like a pharmacist.

The affected individual may now seek information on sources of care for the particular problem. Many of the same sources of communication may be accessed—the Internet, the library, friends and relatives, and health professionals. A surprisingly large number of affected individuals contact their health plans to determine what resources are available for treatment of their condition (and which providers are covered under their plans).

During the next phase (the patient phase), most of the encounters take place at the practitioner's office or other ambulatory care setting. The context for communication has shifted to a more formal setting and information is now transmitted between the symptomatic individual and an authoritative source of information, a physician or other practitioner. The nature of communication may change dramatically at the point the individual is defined as a patient. The communication becomes more one-way and authoritative, reflecting the asymmetric power relationship between provider and patient.

Within the healthcare setting other sources of information come into play. This may involve communication with other health professionals and the dissemination of print materials. Directives may be issued by the physician (and others) to guide the behavior of the patient after the clinical episode.

As discussed elsewhere, communication within the clinical setting with regard to diagnosis, treatment, and subsequent medical regimens is often problematic. The source of information is clearly authoritative and carries the weight of "doctor's orders". However, physicians in particular are not trained in communication methods and research has documented the extent to which adequate information is not transmitted in this context. This defect in the communication process has been held responsible for problems encountered in the management of health problems such as noncompliance with the prescribed regimen, misuse of prescription drugs, and failure to obtain followup care.

search. (There are similarities and differences with other types of consumers in the approach to information search utilized by healthcare consumers.

Initial Awareness.   Awareness refers to the initial exposure of the target population to the good or service being marketed. Thus, during the information search, the healthcare consumer becomes exposed to the various options that exist for addressing the problem at hand.

Knowledge Emergence.   Knowledge concerning the options crystallizes as the healthcare consumer begins to understand the nature of the good or service and appreciate its potential for addressing the problem at hand.

Alternative Evaluation.   At this stage, the consumer is in a position to use the accumulated information to evaluate the available options and make a rational purchase decision. Various options may be ruled out at this point and others maintained in the pool of options.

Contract Assessment.   "Contract assessment" is a step unique to healthcare, in that many goods and services will not be considered for purchase if the provisions of the consumer's insurance plan do not cover them or the available provider does not accept the type of insurance carried (Berkowitz 1996).

Preference Assignment.   Preferences develop at the point that the consumer expresses a tendency for one good or service (e.g., a podiatrist rather than an orthopedic surgeon) and/or decides between different providers of the same service (e.g., Podiatrist A rather than Podiatrist B).

Purchase Decision.   The healthcare consumer makes a decision at this point (or has it made for him) with regard to the good to be purchased or the service to be utilized. Healthcare is different from other consumer contexts in that a variety of players may be involved in the purchase decision at this point.

Product Usage.   At this point the healthcare consumer actually buys the product in question or utilizes the service. This could be as simple as buying Band-Aids at the neighborhood pharmacy or as complex as undergoing a heart transplant.

Post-Purchase Behavior.   This is the stage in the purchase decision process at which consumers take further action after purchase. This involves some type of assessment of the outcomes of the consumption episode and may involve input from family and other parties. Post-purchase behavior involves some assessment of satisfaction with regard to the experience, and the consumer subsequently becomes an advocate for the product or service (or a detractor if dissatisfied).

Virtually every step in the consumer decision-making process has to be modified to allow for the special case of healthcare. While the framework for healthcare decision making is comparable to that for other types of consumers, numerous quirks exist in healthcare that serve to create a unique situation. Familiarity with this process is important for the health professional, and the approach to communicating with the consumer will vary depending on the point in the process at which the consumer is located.

References

Berkowitz, Eric N. 1996. *Essentials of health care marketing.* Gaithersburg, MD: Aspen Publishers.

Berkowitz, Eric N., and Hillestad, Steven G. (1991). *Healthcare marketing plans: From strategy to action.* Boston: Jones and Bartlett.

Eisenberg, D., and R. C. Kessler (1993). Unconventional medicine in the United States. *New England Journal of Medicine,* 328, 246–252.

Fishbein, M., & Ajzen, I. (1975). *Belief, attitude, intention and behavior: An introduction to theory and research.* Reading, MA: Addison-Wesley.

Maslow, Abraham 1970. *Motivation and personality* (2nd ed.). New York: Harper & Row.

National Cancer Institute. (2003). *Making health communication work.* Washington, DC: US Government Printing Office.

National Center for Health Statistics. (2002). *Health United States, 2002.* Washington, DC: US Government Printing Office.

Additional Resources

Bandura, A. (1986). *Social foundations of thought and action: A social cognitive theory.* Englewood Cliffs, NJ: Prentice-Hall.

Bettman, J. R. (1979). *An information processing theory of consumer choice.* Reading, MA: Addison-Wesley.

Beyer, J. M., & Trice, H. M. (1978). *Implementing change: Alcoholism policies in work organizations.* New York: Free Press.

Green, L.W., Gottlieb, N. H., & Parcel, G. S. (1987). Diffusion theory extended and applied. In W. B.Ward (Ed.), *Advances in Health Education and Promotion.* Greenwich, CT: JAI Press.

Janz, N. K., & Becker, M. H. (1984). The health belief model: A decade later. *Health Education Quarterly, 11,* 1–47.

Lefebvre, R. C. (2000). Theories and models in social marketing. In P. N. Bloom & G. T. Gundlach (Eds.), *Handbook of marketing and society.* Thousand Oaks, CA: Sage.

McGuire, W. J. (1984). Public communication as a strategy for inducing health-promoting behavioral change. *Preventive Medicine,* 13(3), 299–313.

Porras, J. I., & Roberston, P. J. (1987). Organization development theory: A typology and evaluation. In R.W.Woodman & W. A. Pasmore (Eds.), *Research in organizational change and development* (Vol. 1). Greenwich, CT: JAI Press.

Prochaska, J. O., & Velicer, W. F. (1997). The transtheoretical model of health behavior change. *American Journal of Health Promotion*, 12(1), 38–48.

Rothman, J., & Tropman, J. E. (1987). Models of community organization and macro practice: Their mixing and phasing. In F. M. Cox, J. L. Ehrlich, J. Rothman, & J. E. Tropman (Eds.), *Strategies of community organization* (4th ed.). Itasca, IL: Peacock.

Rogers, E. M. (1983). *Diffusion of innovations* (3rd ed.). New York: Free Press.

Strecher, V. J., & Rosenstock, I. M. (1997). The health belief model. In K. Glanz, F. M. Lewis, & B. K. Rimer (Eds.), *Health behavior and health education: Theory, research, and practice* (2nd ed.). San Francisco: Jossey-Bass.

Chapter 7

Understanding Communication

U nderstanding the nature of communication and the communication process is critical for the implementation of health communication initiatives. This chapter reviews the various dimensions of communication and discusses their relevance for healthcare. The need to distinguish between communication aimed at individuals, organizations and communities is emphasized. This chapter also discusses the goals of communication and outlines the various steps in the communication process. Critical success factors for effective communication are specified and the barriers to communication discussed.

THE NATURE OF COMMUNICATION

"Communication" involves the transfer of information from a human sender to a human receiver, for the purpose of increasing the receiver's knowledge, enabling him to carry out tasks, or influencing his attitudes and behavior. The "information" transferred refers to the conceptual representation of aspects of a universe in the form of a message that can be encoded and transmitted. Communication in any field may serve a number of purposes. Health communication can be used to:

- Initiate actions
- Make known needs and requirements
- Exchange information, ideas, attitudes or beliefs
- Establish understanding
- Establish and maintain relations

The extent to which a health communication effort serves these purposes depends on the nature of the initiative and the goals that are being pursued.

COMMUNICATION SOURCES

Communication can be generated by a wide variety of sources, and the source is often critical to the acceptability of the message. Sources can be grouped into some major categories and the ones most relevant to health-care are discussed below.

Informal Sources

Much of the information consumers obtain on healthcare is through informal sources, in the form of family, friends and associates. These ad hoc sources of information are important due to their convenience and their credibility. Even today, healthcare consumers point to individuals in these categories as primary sources for health information.

Informal sources may also take the form of social groups, with many consumers obtaining their information concerning health and healthcare in some type of group context. Church groups, social groups or similar groups may provide a context for the effective transfer of information. Indeed, in U.S. society, attitudes toward health and healthcare are more likely to reflect the attitudes of the individual's dominant social groups than of specific individuals.

Formal Sources

Formal sources of health information include those entities that communicate with consumers as part of their job. Formal sources of information generally do not fare well against friends and family. However, in healthcare with its technical dimension, physicians and other providers constitute a primary source of health information. Historically, consumers have placed physicians at the top of the list as their source of health information. Other types of healthcare providers may serve this function, supplemented by the input in many communities of pharmacists.

Other categories of providers such as social workers, psychologists, and counselors maintain as part of their job an information and referral function. Unlike physicians, they may actually be trained in the transfer of information. Some of the information transmission by these providers takes place within group settings in which both the facilitator and the group itself influence the communication process.

All healthcare organizations offer some type of information and, even if they are not in the information business, most healthcare organizations have to make referrals, conveying information in the process. Healthcare organizations are constantly talking to their customers about the who, what, how and where of health services.

Increasingly, consumers report that health plans are a primary source of information on health and healthcare. This is not surprising, since consumers may contact their insurance carrier frequently to determine the level of benefits or the status of their account. With the establishment of provider networks with limited access, health plans have become primary sources of health information.

Impersonal Sources

As mass media became pervasive, an increasing proportion of the population came to receive its information—on healthcare and other topics—from newspapers, magazines, radio and television. These modes of information transfer are the hallmark of modern society, with the Internet now emerging as the king of mass media. The amount of space in both print and electronic media devoted to healthcare has increased dramatically in recent years. Health is a favorite topic of traditional media, and cable television has served to multiply the opportunities for health and healthcare programming. Popular books on healthcare have also become a major source of information on the topic.

While traditional print and electronic media have taken over some of the role of family, friends and even health professionals in the transfer of health-related information, the Internet has become a growing source of information on health and healthcare. Growing numbers of healthcare consumers turn first to the Internet to understand a symptom, find a doctor, or research a pharmaceutical. Despite the sometimes questionable nature of information on the World Wide Web, the Internet is arming consumers with information to take to their physician, pharmacist or other practitioner.

Whatever the source, the effectiveness of a message depends to a large extent on the audience's perception of the source. "Perception" is critical since perceptions rather than reality may determine the manner in which the message is received. The communicator's job is to control and determine the audience's perceptions. Students of communication have identified several dimensions of source credibility (O'Keefe, 1990), listed here in order of their importance:

1. Competence
2. Trustworthiness
3. Goodwill
4. Idealism
5. Similarity

COMPONENTS OF COMMUNICATION

Communication involves a number of components each of which is critical for a successful communication effort. The major components of the communication process are discussed below.

Context

The context is a consideration in the examination of any communication event. The context or environment is the situation in which the communication occurs and includes the physical context, social context, number of people involved, relationship of participants, surrounding events, culture, rituals, and noise.

The physical context is the place in which the communication actually occurs. This could be in the receiver's home, in the workplace, in the physician's office, or any number of other physical settings. The context would be quite different, for example, for preachers delivering a sermon from a pulpit, on the street corner, or over a "televangelism" channel. The temperature, the time of day, nearby people, and any concurrent activities all contribute to the establishment of a context.

The social context represents a major influence on communication. The context may be a group of friends, work associates, or strangers. The context may be familiar or strange. If one were to offer a toast, the approach would be different based on whether the context was the neighborhood pub, your daughter's wedding, or the Nobel Prize award banquet. Such factors as the level of formality, use of appropriate language, familiarity with the audience members, use of humor, content of the message, appropriate dress, and other factors may be influenced by social context.

The context for the transmission of health information is an important consideration. The same information conveyed by the physician in his/her office, around the water fountain at work, from a close family member, or via the Internet will have different degrees of impact. Some contexts are clearly more conducive to the transfer of health-related information than others.

Message

In the communication field, a message represents information that is sent from a source to a receiver. The message includes any thought or idea expressed briefly in a plain or secret language prepared in a form suitable for transmission by any means of communication. The message is the explanation, response, set of instructions, or recommendations that help accomplish the aim of the communication process.

Much of the discussion during the development of a communication initiative focuses on what to say and how to say it. Health communicators must determine what information is to be provided, the style and tone in which it is presented, and what the message must ultimately convey. If the message does not resonate with the target audience, the communication effort is likely to fail.

Channels

Communication occurs through a specific channel or channels. Channels are also referred to as the medium, hence references to "mass media" or to "the media" as a collective term for journalists working in any form of mass media. The channel determines the means in which the communication is delivered and received. Channels differ from each other in terms of attributes, attention getting, and volume of information conveyed, among other factors. A book, for example, has more credibility than television. More information can be communicated in a newspaper article than a television newscast. On the other hand, television has live pictures that make the communication more engaging.

Each type of channel has benefits and drawbacks. Factors to be considered in selecting a channel (and questions to be asked) include:

- The intended audience(s)
  - Will the channel reach and influence the intended audiences?
  - Is the channel acceptable to and trusted by the intended audiences?
- Compatibility with the message
  - Is the channel appropriate for conveying information at the desired level of simplicity or complexity?
  - If skills need to be modeled, can the channel model and demonstrate specific behaviors?
- Channel reach
  - How many people will be exposed to the message through this channel?
  - Can the channel meet intended audience interaction needs?
  - Can the channel allow the intended audience to control the pace of information delivery?
- Cost and accessibility
  - Is this a cost-effective channel given the objectives?
  - Are the resources available to use the channel and the specific activity?
- Activities and materials:
  - Is the channel appropriate for the activity or material you plan to produce?
  - Will the channel and activity reinforce messages and activities you plan through other routes to increase overall exposure among the intended audiences?

(Interactive channels are of increasing importance for health communication and Box 7.1 provides a discussion of these types of channels.)

Box 7.1

Internet and Multimedia Channels

The various types of Internet and multimedia channels are defined
below (in alphabetical order):

CD-ROMs—Computer disks that can contain an enormous amount
of information, including sound and video clips and interactive devices.

Chat rooms—Places on the Internet where users hold live typed
conversations. The "chats" typically involve a general topic. To begin
chatting, users need chat software, most of which can be downloaded
from the Internet for free.

Electronic mail (e-mail)—A technology that allows users to send and
receive messages to one or more individuals on a computer via the
Internet.

Interactive television—Technologies that allow television viewers to
access new dimensions of information (e.g., link to Web sites, order
materials, view additional background information, play interactive
games) through their television during related TV programming.

Internet— A global network connecting millions of computers all over
the world, allowing for the exchange of information; a network of
networks.

Intranets—Electronic information sources with limited access (e.g.,
Web sites available only to members of an organization or employees
of a company). Intranets can be used to send an online newsletter with
instant distribution or provide instant messages or links to sources of
information within an organization.

Kiosks—Displays containing a computer programmed with related information. Users can follow simple instructions to access personally
tailored information of interest and, in some cases, print out what they
find. A relatively common health application involves placing kiosks in
pharmacies to provide information about medicines.

Box 7.1 (Continued).

Mailing lists (listservs)—E-mail-based discussions on a specific topic. All the subscribers to a list can elect to receive a copy of every message sent to the list, or they may receive a regular "digest" disseminated via e-mail.

Newsgroups—Collections of e-mail messages on related topics. The major difference between newsgroups and listservs is that the newsgroup host does not disseminate all the messages the host sends or receives to all subscribers. In addition, subscribers need special software to read the messages. Some newsgroups are regulated (i.e., messages are screened for appropriateness to the topic before they are posted).

Websites—Documents on the World Wide Web that provide information from an organization (or individual) and provide links to other sources of Internet information. Websites give users access to text, graphics, sound, video, and databases. A Website can consist of one Web page or thousands of Web pages.

Timing

People use the expression: "Timing is everything," and that applies especially to communication. Timing can be thought of in a variety of ways. In a mechanical sense, timing could refer to the day of the week or time of the day at which communication occurs. It could also refer to the frequency of exposures established. Radio and television advertising is carefully planned to take advantage of the habits of listeners or viewers, and information is available on the timing that is appropriate for various target audiences. (Public service announcements may be run at 3 a.m. because that is when a timeslot is available that paying advertisers may find unattractive.)

Timing may also refer to the state of readiness on the part of the target audience vis-à-vis the message that is being conveyed. Different audiences are amenable to the receipt of information at different times, not in terms of clock time but in terms of their current situation. It is very difficult, for example, to interest teenagers or young adults in the risk of chronic disease since their age and health status make this an irrelevant topic. Or a woman may only be interested in information on pediatricians around the time that her baby is due to be delivered. It is very difficult to talk about HIV and AIDS within some church settings, and this type of situation is a particular issue in health communication, since many topics are unpleasant or make the recipient uncomfortable.

CHANNEL TYPES AND CHARACTERISTICS

Although informal channels are certainly an important consideration in the study of health communication, this section will focus on formal channels. Formal channels can be categorized in terms of the "level" at which they are focused. They involve communication at the interpersonal, small group, organizational, community, and mass media levels. Each of these will be discussed in turn.

Interpersonal channels involve information transfer by means of counseling sessions, training courses, and "hot line" access. This category would, of course, include informal discussion. Communication at this level has the benefit of a credible source, the opportunity for two-way discussion, and a supportive or even inspirational aspect. The disadvantages of this type of channel include the "cost" involved (for each of the small number of participants), the time involved, and the limited number of consumers who can be reached in this manner.

Organizational and community channels include such contexts as town hall meetings or other community meetings, organizational events, and workplace sessions. This type of channel has the benefit of sponsorship by a credible organization, access to a "captive" audience, relatively low cost, opportunities for sharing experiences among those in similar situations, and the potential to reach a relatively large audience. The drawbacks to this category of channel include the potential for high costs, the impact of organizational constraints, a lack of personal attention for participants, and the potential for the organization to influence the content or nature of the program.

Mass media channels are probably the type of channel that most easily comes to mind when thinking of communication with the public. Common forms of mass media include print forms such as newspapers and magazines and electronic forms such as radio and television. The Internet has become an important new form of mass media, although with obvious differences from other electronic forms of communication.

Newspapers are the most common form of print media and communication in them can take a variety of forms. They offer a vehicle for paid advertisements and promotional inserts. They also offer the opportunity for public relations type communication, in the form of news items, feature stories, op/ed pieces, public service announcements, and even letters to the editor.

Newspapers generally have broad coverage, can allot more space to a health-related topic than electronic media, and, while the papers themselves have limited "shelf life", readers can excerpt articles about a health topic, notices of educational programs, and phone numbers of organizations that are promoting their services.

Newspapers are not without their drawbacks as a vehicle for communication. They represent a "shotgun" approach to communication, and the communicator has no control over who is exposed to the message. While the coverage is potentially very broad, readership of newspapers is steadily declining. In general, the publisher has total control over what is inserted and what an organization may consider newsworthy may not be deemed as such by the newspaper. (There are "community"-type newspapers that may publish submitted articles essentially verbatim.) Finally, newspaper advertising tends to be relatively expensive.

Radio represents the oldest of the electronic media. Much like newspapers, radio stations run advertisements and public service announcements. They also air news reports and may have programming dedicated to health issues. This medium has the advantages of being able to target specific audiences, generate interaction through call-in shows, and offer a wide range of options in terms of timing. Further, radio advertising is a relatively good value compared to other types of advertising and certainly involves lower production costs than television ads.

On the negative side of the ledger, reaching a targeted audience means reaching a smaller audience. Competition for choice air times may be stiff, making the best times expensive. Public service announcements are likely to be aired at odd times when few of the targeted audience may be listening. It is also difficult to preserve information provided via the radio and refer to it later.

By the 1960s television had become the medium of the day and, for many, represents the first choice for communicating a message. Television offers similar opportunities to radio but with the advantage of video, special effects, color, and so forth. Television is driven by advertising and, with the advent of cable television, this medium represents an opportunity to reach as broad or as narrow an audience as desired. Television programming typically includes news programs, and healthcare is certainly a hot topic today. There are many health-related feature programs and, indeed, entire networks developed to health-related topics. Television also offers the opportunity for dramatic programming, using investigative journalism and drama productions to highlight health-related issues. Television stations are also required to run a certain amount of public service announcements.

Communication via television has the advantage of broad reach if desired by means of network coverage or relatively narrow targeting through use of cable stations. The viewing preferences of the intended audience can be exploited and this may be an effective means of reaching low-income audiences who might not be accessible through other forms of communication. The production capabilities associated with television allow for high-impact, emotionally charged programming.

Television does have the disadvantages of high production costs for ads and high placement costs. It may not be possible to place ads at the most desirable times, and public service announcements are likely to be run infrequently and at times of low viewership. More so than other media, television is characterized by communication "clutter", making it extremely difficult to attract attention to a particular effort at communication. As now clearly demonstrated, the ability to retain information transmitted via television is limited, making the window for impacting the targeted audience very narrow.

Findings from the "Healthstyles Survey" conducted by the Centers for Disease Control and Prevention suggest daytime and prime time TV dramas serve a critical health education service when they provide accurate, timely information about disease, injury and disability in their storylines. For U.S. citizens who watch at least a few times a month—particularly for the 43% or 108 million people who are regular viewers, or viewers who watch two or more times a week—popular television series represent an important potential source of health information. Since audience reach is broad and effects are very strong, especially among minority viewers, the shows provide a critical channel for prevention information for these audiences. However, if a show fails to convey accurate information or portrays risky behavior without the associated health consequences, viewers may suffer negative effects as well.

The daily and weekly formats of daytime and prime time TV dramas can be very influential since audiences develop familiarity with regular characters and identify with characters they perceive to be like themselves. Behavioral scientists have demonstrated that this type of identification enhances learning and prevention – because audience members are inclined to model desirable behavior and avoid undesirable behavior – based on the experiences of characters they have come to know. Letters to the shows provide anecdotal evidence about the effects TV entertainment shows have on their audiences. Such letters from viewers include thanks for important health information, report visits and calls to doctors, tell of advice given to friends, and encourage producers to keep up the good work.

In many ways, the Internet is becoming the vehicle of choice for accessing health-related information. As such, it is becoming an increasingly common vehicle for health communicators. The Internet supports the ability to transmit information in a variety of ways, including informative websites, e-mail transmission, chat rooms, and newsgroups. Paid advertising is found on many websites, and some carry public service announcements. Once established, the production costs for additional website material are relatively small. The Internet has the advantage of providing information "on demand" and in whatever form the viewer wants to see it.

The Internet also has the advantages of being instantly updated (think news or sports scores), and can provide live audio and video feeds in the same manner as radio and television. Information can be customized for specific recipients and the content carefully controlled. Further, the Internet offers the opportunity for interaction (e.g., the on-line health risk appraisal) and, the two-way transfer of information provides an advantage over any other form of communication. Unlike any other medium, the Internet serves as a "window" to an unlimited number of other sources of information.

The challenges in developing effective websites are well documented and discussed elsewhere in this text. A poorly developed website may do more harm than good, and the costs involved in developing an adequate site may be high. Time, effort and money must be devoted to maintenance in addition to the original development costs. There is always the danger that Internet penetration is low among the intended audience, and even "wired" consumers may have to develop skills at navigating the site and participating in chat rooms.

THE COMMUNICATION PROCESS

A number of communication models have been developed for application to marketing, and Berkowitz (1996) has adopted one of these for healthcare. While Berkowitz focuses on marketing communication, this model can be readily applied to health communication. An understanding of each of these nine components is important for effective communication.

1. The **sender** is the party sending the message to another party. Also referred to as the communicator or the source, the sender is the "who" of the process and takes the form of a person, company or spokesperson for someone else.
2. The **message** refers to the combination of symbols and words that the sender wishes to transmit to the receiver. This would be considered the "what" of the process and indicates the content that the sender wants to convey.
3. **Encoding** refers to the process of translating the meaning to be transmitted into symbolic form (words, signs, sounds, etc.). At this point a concept is converted into something transmittable.
4. The **channel** refers to the means used to deliver a marketing message from sender to receiver. This indicates the "how" of the process or what connects the sender to the receiver.
5. The **receiver** is the party who receives the message, also known as the audience or the destination. It is the receiver toward whom the communication effort is directed.

6. **Decoding** refers to the process carried out by the receiver when he converts the "symbols" transmitted by the sender into a form that makes sense to him. This process assumes that the receiver is using the same basis for decoding that the sender used for encoding.
7. The **response** refers to the reaction of the receiver to the message. This is the point at which the effect of the message is gauged, and relates to the meaning that the receiver attaches to it.
8. **Feedback** refers to the aspect of the receiver's response that the receiver communicates back to the sender. The type of feedback will depend on the channel, and the effectiveness of the effort is gauged in terms of the feedback.
9. **Noise** refers to any factor that prevents the decoding of a message by the receiver in the way intended by the sender. Noise can be generated by the sender, the receiver, the message, the channel, the environment and so forth.

BARRIERS TO COMMUNICATION

The communication process could be unsuccessful for any number of reasons. Factors that might influence this process include selective attention on the part of the receiver, selective distortion on the part of the receiver (e.g., changing the message to fit preconceptions), selective recall whereby the receiver only absorbs part of the message, and message rehearsal whereby the receiver is reminded by the message of related issues that tend to distract the receiver from the point of the message. Any of the aspects of communication discussed above can have barriers associated with them. These include the source of the information, context, message, channel and/or timing. Although the growing access of the public to interactive media is helping to overcome some of the barriers to communication, many of the barriers noted above remain unaffected by technological solutions to information transfer. Some of the types of barriers are discussed below.

Transmission Barriers

Things that get in the way of message transmission are sometimes called "noise." Communication may be difficult because of noise and associated problems. A bad cellular phone line or a noisy restaurant can inhibit communication. If an E-mail message or letter is not formatted properly, or if it contains grammatical and spelling errors, the receiver may not be able to concentrate on the message because the physical appearance of the letter or E-mail is sloppy and unprofessional.

Conflicting Messages

Messages that cause a conflict in perception for the receiver may result in incomplete communication. For example, if a person constantly uses jargon or slang to communicate with someone from another country who has never heard such expressions, mixed messages are sure to result. Another example of conflicting messages might be if a supervisor requests a report immediately without giving the report writer enough time to gather the proper information. Does the report writer emphasize speed in writing the report or accuracy in gathering the data? A current example of conflicting messages in healthcare involves the debate over the health benefits of moderate alcohol consumption.

Information Overload

In reality, people do not pay attention to all communications they receive but selectively attend to and purposefully seek out information. A received message containing too much information is likely to create a barrier to effective communication. If information is coming too fast and furious, people tend to put up barriers since the amount of information is coming so fast that it becomes difficult to interpret the information. This is an innate trait of human beings and can be seen in a baby that miraculously falls asleep in the face of intrusive attention. If a topic has 25 salient points, it may be possible to only communicate two or three of them at one time; otherwise the receiver is overwhelmed by the avalanche of information.

Channel Barriers

The choice of channel is critical for effective communication and, if a sender chooses an inappropriate channel of communication, insurmountable barriers may be imposed. Detailed instructions presented over the telephone, for example, may be frustrating for both communicators. Some consumer may be so resistant to direct (read "junk") mail, that they refuse to deal with any organization that sends them unsolicited communication in the mail. The credibility (or lack thereof) of a channel will determine the extent to which the message is acceptable to the receiver.

Social and Cultural Barriers

Effective communication with people of different cultures is especially challenging. Cultures provide people with ways of seeing, hearing, and interpreting the world. Thus the same words can mean different things to people from different cultures, even when they talk the "same" language.

When the languages are different, and translation has to be used to communicate, the potential for misunderstandings increases.

Ting-Toomey (1994) describes three ways in which culture interferes with effective cross-cultural understanding. First is what she calls "cognitive constraints." These are the frames of reference or world views that provide a backdrop that all new information is compared to or inserted into. This framework facilities one's interpretation of the information that is transmitted.

Second are "behavior constraints." Each culture has its own rules about proper behavior which affect verbal and nonverbal communication. Whether one looks the other person in the eye or not; whether one says what one means overtly or talks around the issue; and how close the people stand to each other when they are talking are practices that differ from culture to culture.

Ting-Toomey's third factor is "emotional constraints." Different cultures regulate the display of emotion differently. Members of some cultures get very emotional when they are debating an issue. They yell, cry, exhibit their anger, fear, frustration, or other feelings openly. Other cultures try to keep their emotions hidden, exhibiting or sharing only the "rational" or factual aspects of the situation.

Literacy Levels

The literacy level of any target audience must be taken into consideration. *Health literacy* is defined as the ability to read, understand, and act on health information. People of any age, income, race, or background can find it challenging to understand health information. Low health literacy has been identified as a serious barrier to health communication, yet presenting material to well-educated audiences that is well below their level of comprehension can also have a negative affect on the communication process.

The health literacy problem involves more of an issue of understanding medical information rather than one of access to information. In fact, the health of millions of people in the United States may be at risk because of the difficulty some patients experience in understanding and acting on health information.

Medical information is becoming increasingly complex and, all too frequently, physicians do not explain this information in layperson's terms, or in a way that patients can understand. Physicians are under increasing time pressure in today's clinical setting, and they may not even be aware when patients do not understand medical information or instructions. If patients do not understand medication and self-care instructions, a crucial part of their medical care is missing, which may then have an adverse effect on their clinical outcomes. (Literacy levels remain a major barrier to communication in the U.S. healthcare system and this issue is addressed in Box 7.2.)

Box 7.2

Low Health Literacy

Low health literacy—the inability to read, understand, and act on health information—is an emerging public health communication issue that affects people of all ages, races, and income levels. Research shows that most consumers need help understanding healthcare information. Regardless of reading level, patients prefer medical information that is easy to read and understand. For people who don't have strong reading skills, however, easy-to-read healthcare materials are essential.

Limited health literacy increases the disparity in healthcare access among exceptionally vulnerable populations (such as racial/ethnic minorities and the elderly). Low health literacy creates an enormous cost burden on the American healthcare system. Annual health care costs for individuals with low literacy skills are four times higher than those with higher literacy skills. Problems with patient compliance and medical errors may be based on poor understanding of health information. The fact that only about 50% of all patients take medications as directed illustrates the downside of low health literacy.

Patients with low health literacy and chronic diseases, such as diabetes, asthma, or hypertension, have less knowledge of their disease and its treatment and fewer correct self-management skills than literate patients. Patients with low literacy skills face a 50% increased risk of hospitalization, compared with patients who have adequate literacy skills.

Research on literacy levels indicates that people with low literacy:

- Make more medication or treatment errors
- Are less able to comply with treatment regimens
- Lack the skills needed to successfully negotiate the healthcare system
- Are at higher risk for hospitalization than people with adequate literacy skills

APPROACHES TO EFFECTIVE COMMUNICATION

Communications experts indicate that effective communications requires certain attributes. The communication must contain value for the receiver, be meaningful, relevant and understandable, and capable of being transmitted in a few seconds. Further, the communication must lend itself to visual presentation if possible, be relevant to the lives of "real" people, and stimulate the receiver emotionally. It is also important that the communication be interesting, entertaining and stimulating.

Research indicates that effective health promotion and communication initiatives adopt an audience-centered perspective, with promotion and communication activities reflecting audiences' preferred formats, channels, and contexts. These considerations are particularly relevant for racial and ethnic populations, who may have different languages and sources of information. In these cases, public education campaigns must be conceptualized and developed by individuals with specific knowledge of the cultural characteristics, media habits, and language preferences of intended audiences. Direct translation of health information or health promotion materials should be avoided. Credible channels of communication need to be identified for each major group. Television and radio channels serving specific racial and ethnic populations can be effective means of delivering health messages when care is taken to account for the language, culture, and socioeconomic situations of the intended audiences.

An audience-centered perspective also reflects the realities of people's everyday lives and their current practices, attitudes and beliefs, and lifestyles. Some specific audience characteristics that are relevant include gender, age, education and income levels, ethnicity, sexual orientation, cultural beliefs and values, primary language(s), and physical and mental functioning. Additional considerations include their experience with the healthcare system, attitudes toward different types of health problems, and willingness to use certain types of health services. Particular attention should be paid to the needs of underserved audience members. (See Box 7.3 for a discussion of the attributes of effective health communication.)

Box 7.3

Attributes of Effective Health Communication

According to documents produced by the Department of Health and Human Services to support the Healthy People 2010 initiative, there are several attributes of effective communication. These are:

- *Accuracy*. The content is valid and free from errors of fact, interpretation or judgment.
- *Availability*. The content is delivered or placed where the audience can access it.

Box 7.3 (Continued).

- *Balance.* Where appropriate, the content presents the benefits and risks of potential actions or recognizes different and valid perspectives on the issue.
- *Consistency.* The content remains internally consistent over time and is consistent with information from other sources.
- *Cultural Competence.* The design, implementation and evaluation processes take into account special issues for select population groups as well as their educational levels.
- *Evidence Based.* Relevant scientific evidence that has undergone comprehensive review and rigorous analysis to formulate practice guidelines, performance measures, review criteria, and technology assessments is included.
- *Reach.* The content gets to or is available to the largest possible number of people in the target population.
- *Reliability.* The source of the content is credible and the content itself is kept up to date.
- *Repetition.* The delivery of/access to the content is continued or repeated over time, both to reinforce the impact with a given audience and to reach new generations.
- *Timeliness.* The content is provided or is available when the audience is most receptive to, or most in need of, the specific information.
- *Understandability.* The reading or language level and format are appropriate for the target audience.

Source: U.S. Department of Health and Human Services (2001). *Healthy People 2010.* Washington, DC: U.S. Government Printing Office.

These factors indicate the complexity involved in the development of effective health communication. One of the main challenges in the design of effective health communication programs is to identify the optimal contexts, channels, content, and reasons that will motivate people to pay attention to and use health information.

References

Berkowitz, Eric. (1996). *Essentials of health care marketing.* Gaithersburg, MD: Aspen.
Daniel O'Keefe. (1990). *Persuasion: Theory and research.* Newbury Park, CA: Sage.
Ting-Toomey, Stella. (Ed.) (1994). *Challenge of facework: Cross-cultural and interpersonal issues.* Albany, NY: State University of New York Press.

Additional Resources

Ad Hoc Committee on Health Literacy for the Council on Scientific Affairs, American Medical Association. (1999). Health literacy: Report of the council on scientific affairs. *JAMA*, 281, 552–557.

Baker, D. W., Parker, R. M., Williams, M. V., et al. (1996). The health care experience of patients with low literacy. *Arch Fam Med*, 5, 329–334.

Baker, D. W., Parker, R. M., Williams, M. V., Clark, W. S. (1998). Health literacy and the risk of hospital admission. *J Gen Intern Med*, 1998, 13, 791–798.

Doak C. C., Doak L. G, Root J. H. (1996). The literacy problem. in *Teaching patients with low literacy skills.* (2nd ed.). Philadelphia: J. B. Lippincott Co.

Pfizer. What is health literacy?: Scope and impact. URL: http://pfizerhealthliteracy.com/whatis.html. Accessed on 1/25/05

Weiss, B. D. (ed.) (1999). *20 common problems in primary care.* New York: McGraw Hill.

Williams, M. V., Baker, D. W., Honig, E. G., Lee, T. M., Nowlan, A. (1998). Inadequate literacy is a barrier to asthma knowledge and self-care. *Chest*, 114, 1008–1015.

Chapter 8

Steps in the Health Communication Process

T he health communication process can be complicated, but like any complex process the health communication effort can be broken down into a number of discrete steps. By developing an understanding of these steps the process can become infinitely more manageable. The sections below outline the various steps involved—from beginning to end—in the process. While they are presented in fairly strict sequence, it should be realized that there are situations in which the sequence might be changed or, in rare circumstances, a step be eliminated.

STAGES IN THE HEALTH COMMUNICATION PROCESS

The health communication process can be divided into several distinct stages. For our purposes, we can consider these stages as: planning, development, implementation, and evaluation. Each of these stages will be discussed in turn.

The Planning Stage

Planning is critical to the development of an effective health communication project. A carefully devised plan will enable the project to produce meaningful results. Taking the time to carefully plan the project will ultimately save time by defining program objectives and indicating steps for meeting those objectives.Even if the project is part of a broader health promotion effort, a plan specific to the communication component is necessary.

Indeed, any health communication effort should fit within the context of the organization's overall marketing plan and be informed by its strategic plan. There are some formal planning techniques that have been developed for healthcare and one of them is described in Box 8.1.)

Box 8.1

The PRECEDE-PROCEED Methodology

Once health communication planners identify a health problem, they can use a planning framework such as PRECEDE-PROCEED. This planning system can help identify the social science theories most appropriate for understanding the problem or situation.

Using planning systems like PRECEDE-PROCEED increases the odds of program success by examining health and behavior at multiple levels. Planning systems may emphasize changing people, their environment, or both.

PRECEDE-PROCEED Framework

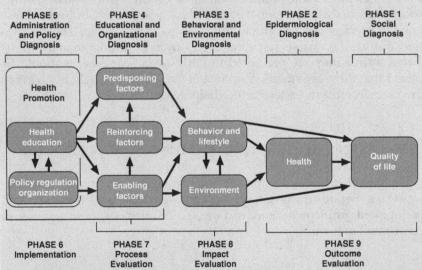

The PRECEDE-PROCEED framework involves an approach to planning that examines the factors contributing to behavior change. These include:

- *Predisposing factors*—the individual's knowledge, attitudes, behavior, beliefs, and values before intervention that affect willingness to change

Box 8.1 (Continued).

- *Enabling factors*—factors in the environment or community of an individual that facilitate or present obstacles to change
- *Reinforcing factors*—the positive or negative effects of adopting the behavior (including social support) that influence continuing the behavior

These factors require that individuals be considered in the context of their community and social structures, and not in isolation, when planning communication or health education strategies. The graphic on the previous page illustrates the PRECEDE-PROCEED model.

Source: National Cancer Institute (2003). *Making health communication work.* Washington: U.S. Government Printing Office.

Stating the Problem or Issue

Defining the problem or the issue is the critical first step in the plan development process. It involves identifying the "real" issues at hand and the specific information required for the development of the communication initiative. Unless the issue is properly defined, the chances of developing a successful campaign are low. Time spent initially isolating the issues represents a good investment.

Stating Assumptions

One of the critical steps at the outset is the stating of assumptions. "Assumptions" are the understandings that drive the planning process, and, if they are not specified early in the process, the communication team may find itself well down the road holding conflicting notions of what the project is really about. Assumptions can relate to demographic trends, reimbursement practices, and any number of other aspects of the healthcare system. Assumptions also should be made about the audience that is being targeted. These would include assumptions related to the nature of the population, the political climate, other options for services, and so forth.

Some assumptions can–and should–be stated at the outset of the planning process. Others will be developed as information is collected and more in-depth knowledge is gained concerning the community, its healthcare needs, and its resources. Although assumptions will undoubtedly be refined as the planning process continues, it is important to begin with at least general assumptions identified.

Reviewing Available Data

Gaps in available information should be noted and sources of additional information identified. The types of sources of information will be determined by the type of issue being addressed in the communication project. The types of information that should be compiled at this stage include:

- The incidence or prevalence of the health problem
- The characteristics of those affected by the identified problem
- The consequences of the health problem for individuals, communities and even the healthcare system
- The possible causes for the condition
- The possible solutions, treatments, or interventions

Both published and unpublished reports may be available from internal and external sources. A number of federal health information clearinghouses and Websites provide information, products, materials, and sources of further assistance for specific health subjects. A helpful first step in assessing the problem may be to access the appropriate Websites and relevant health agencies to obtain information on the health issue being addressed.

It is seldom necessary to "reinvent the wheel" in a world where there is virtually nothing new under the sun. Therefore, it is useful to identify other organizations that are addressing the same issue and determine the types of communication initiatives they have underway. These organizations can indicate what they have learned through the process, provide insights into what works and doesn't work, warn of pitfalls in addressing the issue in question, and even offer collaborative support.

It may be that the data that has been gathered does not give enough insight into the health problem, its resolution, or knowledge about those who are affected in order to proceed. In other instances, there may be enough information to define the problem, specify who is affected, and identify the steps that can resolve it, while other important information about the affected populations is unavailable or outdated.

Sometimes it is impossible to find sufficient information about the problem in question. This may be because the health problem has not yet been well defined. In this case, it might be decided that a communication campaign is an inappropriate response to that particular problem until more becomes known.

Too often health professionals rely on communication alone and set unrealistic expectations for what it can accomplish. It is vitally important to identify all of the components necessary to bring about the desired change and then to carefully consider which of these components is being—or can be—addressed. It is important to determine at this stage what it is about the problem that is amenable to change.

Conducting Additional Research

Research into intended audiences' culture, lifestyle, behaviors and motivations, interests, and needs is a key component to a health communication program's success. As noted in Chapter 6 on communication audiences, an understanding of the target population would include information on demographics, lifestyles, health status, and health behavior—as well as information on the channels, messages, and timing appropriate for the target audience. In some cases, primary research may be required to gather the requisite information for developing a campaign. A number of options are available for conducing primary research and numerous guides are available for consultation.

Most programs use more than one research method. For example, conducting exploratory focus groups with an intended audience at the start of program planning can orient the health communicator to the types of approaches, messages, and channels that are most likely to be successful with a particular group. In some cases, focus groups might be augmented with in-depth interviews to learn more about intended audience members' motivations.

Defining Communication Objectives

Defining communication objectives will help set priorities among possible communication activities and determine the message and content required for each. Once communication objectives have been defined and circulated, they serve as a kind of contract or agreement about the purpose of the communication and establish the types of outcomes to be measured.

Objectives refer to the specific targets to be reached in support of goal attainment. While goals are general statements, objectives should be very specific and stated in clear and concise terms. Any concepts referenced in an objective must be operationalizable and measurable. Objectives must also be time bound, with clear deadlines established for their accomplishment. Finally, they must be amenable to evaluation. In the case of communication initiatives, the objectives should be reasonable and reachable and clearly related to the change desired.

Objectives are stated in such terms as: The rate of teen pregnancy in the community will be reduced from 15 percent to 10 percent by the end of 2005 (in support of the goal of improving the reproductive health of the community). Or, the hospital's orthopedic practice will recruit a sports medicine specialist within the next twelve months (in support of the stated goal of expanding the organization's orthopedic product lines).

It is important to create achievable objectives, and many communication efforts "fail" because the original objectives were unreasonable. It is virtually impossible, for example, to increase a hospital's market share in a major market by more than a couple of percentage points, and any higher goal should be considered unrealistic. If a numerical goal for a particular objective is to be specified, an epidemiologist or statistician can help determine recent rates of change related to the issue to provide guidance for deciding how much change a program can reasonably be expected to effect. Fear of failure should not prevent the setting of measurable objectives. Without them, there is no way to demonstrate that a program has succeeded or is making progress along the way.

Several objectives may be specified related to the goal of a communication initiative. Four or five would not be uncommon, although many more than that become unwieldy (especially if more than one goal is being considered). The objectives should be reviewed by any appropriate parties and possibly by some outside the organization such as experts on the local healthcare system.

Realistically Assessing the Health Communication Approach

In some cases, health communication alone may accomplish little or nothing without policy, technological, or infrastructure changes. In some instances, effective solutions may not yet exist for a communication program to support. For example, no treatment may exist for an illness, or a solution may require services that are not yet available. In these cases, the health communication program should be redirected to support the importance of research on this issue.

Raising awareness or increasing knowledge among individuals or the organizations that serve them is often easily accomplished through the communication process. However, accomplishing such an objective may not necessarily lead to behavior change. For example, it is unreasonable to expect communication to cause a sustained change in complex behaviors or compensate for a lack of health services, products, or resources. The ability and willingness of the intended audience to make certain changes also affect the reasonableness of various communication objectives.

Profiling the Intended Audience(s)

The identification of the intended populations for a program starts with a review of the epidemiology of the problem. This effort will determine who is most affected, who is at the greatest risk, and what other factors contribute to the problem. Intended populations are often defined very broadly, using just a few descriptors (e.g., women over age 50).

Intended audiences are often carved out of these broad population groups and defined more narrowly based on characteristics such as attitudes, demographics, geographic region, or patterns of behavior. Examples might include physically inactive adolescents, heavy smokers with low education and income levels who are fatalistic about health issues, or urban African-American men with hypertension who live in the South. Because the intended audience's ability and willingness to make a behavior change affects the extent to which communication objectives are reasonable and realistic, it is most efficient to select intended audiences and develop communication objectives in tandem.

Formulating a Strategy

At some point during this process, the choice of strategy must be considered. The strategy refers to the generalized approach to communication that is to be taken in response to the challenges identified. This may mean choosing between a public health approach, a free market approach, an educational model, or a public/private consortium approach, to name a few. Any one of these could be thought of as the basis for a strategy and serve as the framework for subsequent communication planning. The strategy should provide overall direction for the initiative, fit the available resources, minimize resistance, reach the appropriate targeted groups, and, ultimately, accomplish the goals of the communication initiative.

While the precise strategic approach to be taken may not be specified at this point, at least the options can be narrowed. This will serve to focus subsequent planning activities by eliminating strategies that are considered unproductive. For example, it may have been determined that the target population must be educated on the issues prior to attempting behavioral change. In this case, the strategy would focus—initially at least—on education and information dissemination.

In another case, initial research may have indicated that a hard-to-reach population is not likely to be easily influenced by standard communication approaches. Here, a strategy that involves partnerships with churches and other organizations in the community that reaches the target audience "where they live" might become important.

Clearly, that planning approach will be quite different than if facility regulation was the focus. Similarly, if a hospital determines, based on available data, that it cannot compete head on with the major player in the market area, its adoption of a "second fiddle" or "flanking" strategy will channel planning in a different direction than if a more confrontational approach was chosen.

A communication strategy should include everything one needs to know to communicate with the intended audience. It defines the intended audience, identifies the actions its members should take, tells how they will benefit (from their perspective, not necessarily from a public health perspective), and how they can most effectively be reached.

Developing the strategy statement provides a good test of whether the project has enough information to begin developing messages. It also gives the communication team an opportunity to obtain management and partner buy-in for the approach. Having an approved strategy statement will save time and effort later. The statement provides both a foundation and boundaries for the materials to be produced and the activities to be implemented.

Choosing the Type of Appeal

There are a variety of ways in which to capture the intended audience's attention. Appeals might be made to their emotions, their intellect, or their pocketbooks. The best approach depends on the nature of the intended audience's preferences, the type of information being communicated and, ultimately, what the project hopes to accomplish. In any case, the choice of type of appeal should reflect the strategy that has been chosen. Examples of types of appeals include the following:

Positive emotional appeals show the benefits intended audience members will gain when they take the action portrayed in the message. Research has shown that, in general, messages that present a major benefit but do not address any drawbacks tend to be most appropriate when intended audience members are already in favor of an idea or practice. In contrast, messages that present a major benefit and directly address any major drawbacks work best when people are not favorably predisposed.

Humorous appeals can work for simple messages, especially if most competing communication is not humorous. The humor should be appropriate for the health issue and convey the main message; otherwise, people tend to remember the joke but not the message. Also, humorous messages can become irritating if repeated too frequently.

Threat (or fear) appeals have been shown to be effective with two groups. Such appeals tend to be more effective with "copers" (people who are not anxious by nature) and "sensation seekers" (certain youth), and when exposure to the message is voluntary (e.g., picking up a brochure rather than mandatory attendance at a substance abuse prevention program). The most appropriate type of appeal may differ from this general guidance, depending upon gender, age, ethnicity, severity of the problem, and the intended audience's relationship to the problem.

Once a communication strategy has been established, all program elements should be compatible with it. This means every program task should contribute to reaching the established objectives and be designed to reach the identified intended audiences; all messages and materials should incorporate the benefits and other information from the strategy statement.

As more is learned about the intended audiences and their perceptions, it may be necessary to alter or refine the strategy statement. However, it should be changed only to reflect information that will strengthen the project's ability to reach its communication objectives.

The Development Stage

Once the planning has been carried out, the emphasis shifts to the development stage. Important aspects of project development are discussed below.

Materials Development

Developing and pretesting messages and materials are important because they indicate early in the process which messages will be most effective with the intended audiences. Knowing this will save time and money. Positive results from pretesting can also generate early buy-in from others in the organization. It is beneficial to start with existing materials, if possible, and determine what may be appropriate for the particular project rather than reinventing the wheel.

Although message and materials development and production are often time consuming and costly, this represents a critical step in the development of a health communication program. Given the magnitude of this task, existing communication materials (booklets, leaflets, posters, public service announcements, videotapes) should be inventoried. If not directly applicable, they may serve as a foundation for subsequent materials development. Or, it may be possible to find existing materials available from health departments, voluntary health organizations, health professional associations, and other sources. Materials produced by the National Institutes of Health, the Centers for Disease Control and Prevention, or other agencies in the U.S. Department of Health and Human Services are often very helpful, and work commissioned by NIH has informed much of this text. Using the communication strategy statement as a guide, the following questions should be posed with regard to any existing materials:

- Are the messages accurate, current, complete, and relevant?
- Are the materials appropriate for the intended audience in terms of format, style, cultural considerations, and readability level?
- Are the materials likely to meet the communication objectives?

Once message concepts have been established for the intended audience, the material formats (e.g., brochure, videotape) that will best suit the project should be determined. These materials should be evaluated in terms of:

- The nature of the message (e.g., its complexity, sensitivity, style)
- The function of the message (e.g., to call attention to an issue or to teach a new skill)
- The activities and channels previously selected
- The budget and other available resources

The development of new materials typically represents a major expenditure. Formats should be chosen that the program can afford. It is important to avoid overspending on materials production in order to afford sufficient quantities, distribution expenses, and process evaluation. Knowledge of the intended audience should be used to combine, adapt, and devise new ways to get the message across. Input should be sought from the intended audience or partners with regard to decisions about materials.

Box 8.2

Concept Testing

Concepts can be presented for testing in a number of ways. The key is to convey the major characteristics of the appeal along with the action the program wants intended audiences to take and the benefit they will receive as a result. (Marketing experts have developed a number of techniques for concept testing and their skills should be utilized.) This process typically involves initially testing the message, testing draft materials incorporating the message, and testing final materials before they are sent to production.

Once the intended audiences have been defined and communication strategies developed, testing the concepts with intended audiences can help determine message appeals (e.g., fear-arousing versus factual), spokespersons (e.g., a scientist, public official, or member of the intended audience), and language (determined by listening to research participants' language). Testing is especially important if the program deals with a new issue, because it will help you understand where the issue fits within the larger context of the intended audience's life and perceptions. Messages and materials should be pretested in a context that approximates "real life." Theater-style testing, for example, can approximate reality, using a simulated television-viewing environment. Using

Box 8.2 (Continued).

multiple methods can help ensure the development of an accurate picture of the intended audience members and their likely responses to the program.

Concept testing will help save the program time and money because it will identify which messages work best with intended audiences. Use concept testing to identify:

- Which concept has the strongest appeal and potential for effect
- Confusing terms or concepts
- Language used by the intended audience
- Weaker concepts that should be eliminated
- New concepts

Message concept tests often ask participants to rank a group of concepts from most to least compelling and then to explain their rankings. Participants then discuss benefits and problems associated with each concept. Health communicators often use a sentence or brief paragraph to describe a concept to participants. For example, the following are two "don't smoke" concepts for teens:

1. Smoking harms your appearance.
2. Cigarette advertisers have created a myth that smoking makes a person more attractive. They're lying.

While both concepts address attractiveness, the first concept uses it as the focal point of a negative appeal (to avoid becoming less attractive, don't smoke), whereas the second concept uses a factual approach and a different benefit—avoid being manipulated by the tobacco industry—designed to appeal to teens' strong desire not to be manipulated.

In each of the concepts above, both the action the intended audience members should take and the benefit are implied, not stated. This approach works in situations where the desired behavior is obvious. In other situations, the behavior or the benefit will need to be mentioned.

Source: National Cancer Institute (2003). *Making health communication work.* Washington: U.S. Government Printing Office.

Planning and Launch

Before the launch of a communication initiative, it is important to plan for distribution, promotion, and process evaluation. This requires the communication staff to develop a launch plan, produce sufficient quantities of materials, and prepare for subsequent tasks. The nature of the project might benefit from a quiet, low-key launch, or its nature may mandate a major kick-off event. A kickoff event can create broader awareness of the program and promote community involvement. Kickoff events are an excellent way to develop relationships with people who may be willing to get involved in the program. Scheduling an event also creates a deadline, which will help the program avoid unnecessary lag time or protracted preparations.

In order to enhance media coverage for a kickoff event, a number of steps can be taken. For example, the organization might create a news "hook" or angle that makes the event newsworthy, inform the media of the event in a timely manner, create media kits to facilitate accurate reporting of the issue, and include the full range of appropriate media. These would include specialized media, such as community newspapers, cable TV stations, radio, health-related publications (the trade press), foreign-language publications or broadcast media, Internet "zines" and Web sites, and organization publications. These media may have a greater incentive to use a feature story or news item than general newspapers or regular TV stations, and they can ensure an audience at a press conference if the mainstream media don't show up.

The Implementation Stage

Planning is ultimately only an exercise, albeit a meaningful one. The payoff comes in the implementation of the plan. The planning process creates a road map which the communication staff uses to move the initiative to where it needs to be. It is during the implementation stage, however, that the process often breaks down. The oft-repeated maxim that "the last plan is still sitting on the shelf" generally reflects a failure in implementation rather than any flaw in the plan itself.

Transitioning to Development

The transition from planning to implementation involves a hand-off from the planning team to the management team. Implementation must occur at several different levels and within different sectors of the community or divisions of the organization. For this reason, the implementation of the plan requires a level of coordination that few organizations have in place.

In order to approach plan implementation systematically, the communications team should develop both a detailed project plan and an implementation matrix. An implementation matrix can be developed using a spreadsheet and should lay out who is to do what and when they are to do it. The matrix should list every action called for by the plan, breaking each action down into tasks, if appropriate. For each action or task the responsible party should be identified, along with any secondary parties that should be involved in this activity. The matrix should indicate resource requirements (in terms of staff time, money and other resources). The start and end dates for this activity should be identified. Any prerequisites for accomplishing this task should be identified at the outset and factored into the project plan. Finally, benchmarks should be established that allow the planning team to determine when the activity has been completed.

The nature of the progress indicators used will be determined by the type of plan. In many cases, *operational* benchmarks will be important. These may relate to utilization levels, facility development, or staffing changes, as well as others. *Clinical* standards may be established in many cases as well. These may focus on outcomes such as a reduction in the hospital mortality rate or improvement in surgical outcomes. *Financial* benchmarks are likely to be included in many plans. The success of communication initiatives will often be measured in terms of such factors as revenue, profit, or return on investment.

A master schedule should be established for development, implementation, and evaluation activities. The schedule should include every possible task from initial planning to project completion. The resource requirements from the implementation matrix should be combined to determine total project resource requirements. The timetable should be considered a flexible management tool to be reviewed and updated regularly.

Managing the Campaign

The primary tasks involved in managing a health communication campaign include monitoring activities, staff, and budget; problem solving; process evaluation; measuring audience response; and revising plans and operations. The plan developed to manage the campaign should indicate how and when resources will be needed, when specific events will occur, and at what points you will assess your efforts. On-going process evaluation will determine the extent to which activities are being completed at scheduled times, the intended audiences are being reached, which activities or materials are most successful, and which aspects of the program need to be altered or eliminated.

It is often possible to correct problems quickly if they can be identified. For example, if the public is being asked to call you for more information, a simple form (electronic or manual) for telephone operators to use to record the questions asked and the answers given would be useful if not essential. Any project of this type should be monitored to review responses for inquiry patterns, assure that correct or adequate information is being given, and determine whether more or different information may be needed.

Determining the Channels

Message delivery channels have changed significantly in recent years (National Cancer Institute, 2003). Today, channels are more numerous, are often more narrowly focused on an intended audience, and represent changes that have occurred in healthcare delivery, the mass media, and society.

Interpersonal channels (e.g., physicians, friends, family members, counselors, parents, clergy, and coaches of the intended audiences) put health messages in a familiar context. These channels are more likely to be trusted and influential than media sources. Developing messages, materials, and links into interpersonal channels may require time; however, these channels are among the most effective, especially for affecting attitudes, skills, and behavior/behavioral intent. Influence through interpersonal contacts may work best when the individual is already familiar with the message, for example, from hearing it through mass media exposure. (Similarly, mass media are most effective at changing behavior when they are supplemented with interpersonal channels.)

Group channels (e.g., brown bag lunches at work, classroom activities, church group discussions, neighborhood gatherings, and club meetings) can help an initiative more easily reach a larger share of the intended audience while retaining some of the influence of interpersonal channels. Health messages can be designed for groups with specific things in common, such as workplace, school, church, club affiliations, or favorite activities, and these channels add the benefits of group discussion and affirmation of the messages. As with interpersonal channels, working through group channels can require significant levels of effort. Influence through group channels is more effective when groups are already familiar with the message from interpersonal channels.

The Evaluation Stage

The notion of evaluating the communication project should be top of mind on the first day of the process, and the means for evaluation should be built into the process itself. Evaluation is necessary to determine the efficiency of the process and the effectiveness of the initiative. Evaluation techniques focus to two types of analysis: process (or formative) analysis and outcome (or summative) analysis. The former evaluates systems, procedures, communication processes, and other factors that contribute to the efficient operation of a program. Outcome evaluation focuses more on end results or what is ultimately accomplished. Process evaluation essentially measures efficiency, while outcome evaluation measures effectiveness (Adams and Schvaneveldt, 1991).

Evaluation should involve on-going monitoring of the communication process, including benchmarks and/or milestones for assessment along the way. This will require the clarification of the objectives and goals of the initiative. According to the Community Tool Box (developed by the University of Kansas), the following issues should be addressed during the evaluation process:

- *Planning and implementation issues*: How well was the program or initiative planned out, and how well was that plan put into practice?
- *Assessing attainment of objectives:* How well has the program or initiative met its stated objectives?
- *Impact on participants*: How much and what kind of a difference has the program or initiative made for its targets of change?
- *Impact on the community:* How much and what kind of a difference has the program or initiative made on the community as a whole?

Data collection and benchmarking are extremely important for measuring progress in meeting objectives, and documenting the process of change is an ongoing task that should occur on a regular basis. Health communicators should submit updates to the key parties involved in the initiative.

Once the questions to be answered through the evaluation have been identified, the next step is to decide which methods will best address those questions. Some of the methods to be utilized include: a monitoring and feedback system; member surveys about the initiative; goal attainment report; behavioral surveys; interviews with key participants; and community-level indicators of impact.

Although evaluation techniques are often praised for their bottom-line objectivity, they are also useful in healthcare where it is not possible to place a dollar value on everything. Thus, cost-effectiveness analysis can take into consideration the intangible aspects of the communication initiative in its evaluation. Thus, strict cost/benefit analyses are likely to be less suitable for use in healthcare than in most other industries.

References

Adams, G. R. and Schvaneveldt. J. D. (1991). *Understanding research methods.* New York: Congman.

National Cancer Institute. (2003). *Making health communication work.* Washington: US Government Printing Office.

University of Kansas. (N.D.) Community tool box. Web-based planning guide. URL: http://ctb.lsi.ukans.edu.

Additional Resources

Academy for Educational Development. (1995). *A tool box for building health communication capacity*. Washington, DC.

Andreasen, A. (1995). *Marketing social change: Changing behavior to promote health, social development, and the environment*. San Francisco: Jossey-Bass.

Calvert, P. (Ed.). (1996). *The communicator's handbook: Tools, techniques, and technology* (3rd ed.). Gainesville, FL: Maupin House.

Green, L. W., & Kreuter, M. W. (1999). *Health promotion planning: An educational and ecological approach* (3rd ed.). Mountain View, CA: Mayfield.

Green, L. W., & Ottoson, J. M. (1999). *Community and population health* (8th ed.). New York: McGraw-Hill.

Thomas, Richard K. (2003). *Health services planning*. New York: Kluwer.

Chapter 9

Traditional Approaches to Health Communication

C hapter 9 reviews the "traditional" techniques applied to health communication, emphasizing the need to apply different approaches to different targets in different situations. These approaches may involve simple initiatives (e.g., information and referral) or complex endeavors (e.g., behavioral change initiatives). The use of the various forms of media is described and the pros and cons of various media are discussed.

TRADITIONAL COMMUNICATION TECHNIQUES

The following methods for communicating are for the most part long established in healthcare. The characteristics of each are discussed, along with their relative merits for communicating health information.

Distribution of Materials

While the distribution of materials is not a technique in the same sense as advertising or telemarketing, it provides the backbone of much of what is considered health communication. The development and distribution of brochures, self-help guides, and health education materials is one of the common denominators of most forms of health communication. While the distribution of materials may not be the main form of exposure for certain health programs, it is likely to be a component of most initiatives. If, for example, a health fair serves as a vehicle for exposing the public to a healthcare issue or service, materials will invariably be distributed.

119

Print materials have long been the staple of health communication, but these are increasingly being supplemented by audio and video materials as the decreasing cost of technology have made these formats more feasible. And, now, the Internet has become a major outlet for distributing electronic "brochures". (The Internet as a communication tool is addressed in the next chapter.)

Information and Referral •

An important function of many organizations is information and referral. Indeed, some organizations exist solely for the purpose of providing information on healthcare programs and directing individuals to the appropriate services. This type of information transfer may be provided in person (e.g., via a case manager), by telephone (e.g., the use of a "hotline"), or by mail. Information and referral is probably the most straightforward of the communication techniques, although, as will be seen, this function has been carried to new levels with the advent of ask-a-nurse programs and other triage services. The Internet is fast becoming a major venue for information and referral activities.

Public Relations

"Public relations" (PR) is a form of communication management that seeks to make use of publicity and other non-paid forms of promotion and information to influence feelings, opinions or beliefs about an organization and its services. Public relations may involve press releases, press conferences, distribution of feature stories to the media, public service announcements and other publicity-oriented activities.

In the past, healthcare organizations often utilized public relations for crisis management and damage control, justifying controversial actions, explaining negative events, and so forth. Over time, however, public relations has been cast in a more proactive light as healthcare organizations have come to appreciate the benefits of a strong PR program. Despite the emergence of contemporary forms of communication involving advanced technology, public relations remains a staple of most healthcare organizations. (See Box 9.1 for a discussion of the use of press conferences.)

The public service announcement (PSA) has become a staple of many not-for-profit organizations in healthcare. Unpaid placements in newspapers, radio and television can provide extensive exposure to a service, organization or cause. Some forms of media are required to run public service announcements and others may be glad to do it. Although there are no costs associated with the placement, there are expenses involved in production

Box 9.1

Holding a Press Conference

Health communication initiatives often involve a press conference. Since a health communication program launch is unlikely to get much media attention if the program simply calls a press conference, attracting the media requires a dedicated effort. Tying the program's launch to important health news can help. Such news could include announcing the results of a recent health study, releasing new statistics on the topic, or announcing the start of a comprehensive or multi-organization health program of which your program is a part. Even more attractive is announcing such news *plus* having representatives of the intended audience or other individuals tell compelling personal stories.

In order to hold a successful press conference, health communicators should:

- Be realistic about the media invited.
- Decide who will announce which aspects of the news.
- Schedule the press conference at a time for the best exposure *and* in keeping with the media's needs (e.g., news deadlines).
- Assign a staff person to arrange a suitable room and any equipment needed.
- Deliver the news release or press kit in person to key reporters who didn't attend the press conference.

(especially for a high-cost medium like television), and the organization has little influence over the physical placement or listening/viewing time placement for radio and television.

Another application of public relations is "media advocacy". Media advocacy involves the strategic use of mass media as a resource for advancing a social or public policy initiative. It is an important, and often essential, part of social action and advocacy campaigns because the media highlight public concerns and spur public action. Effective media advocacy involves developing an understanding of how an issue relates to prevailing public opinion and values and designing messages that frame the issues to maximize their impact.

Preparatory to a press conference, it is usually helpful to develop a media kit. (This might also be done to support other types of communication efforts such as advertising.) A media kit would include a press conference agenda, press release, background information on the issue (including fact sheets), biographies of the speakers, program materials and contact information.

Formal Communication Functions

Large healthcare organizations typically establish mechanisms for communicating with their various publics (both internal and external). Communications staff develop materials for dissemination to the public and the employees of the organization. Internal newsletters and publications geared to relevant customer groups (e.g., patients, enrollees) are generated, and patient education materials are frequently developed by communications staff. Separate communication departments may be established or this function may overlap with the public relations or community outreach functions.

Print was the medium of choice for communication throughout the 1960s in spite of the increasingly influential role the electronic media were playing for marketers in other industries. Annual reports, informational brochures, and publications targeted to the community continue to be standard products of communication departments.

Community Outreach

Community outreach is a vehicle for communication that seeks to present the programs of the organization to the community and establish relationships with community organizations. Community outreach may involve episodic activities such as health fairs or educational programs for community residents. This function may also include on-going initiatives involving outreach workers who are visible within the community on a recurring basis. This aspect of marketing emphasizes the organization's commitment to the community and its support of community organizations. While the benefits of community outreach activities are not as easily measured as some more direct marketing activities, the organization often gains customers as a result of its health screening activities, followup from educational seminars, or outreach worker referrals.

One objective of community outreach initiatives is to generate word-of-mouth communication (WOM) concerning the organization or its services. WOM communication occurs when people share information about products or promotions with friends and associates. Efforts to generate positive word-of-mouth support are important since there is often a tendency for WOM communication to be negative.

Pursuant to community outreach programs, information might be disseminated in the form of educational materials, lectures, and person-to-person interaction. Community outreach could involve public forums or privately sponsored programs.

Government Relations

Many healthcare organizations have a long history of government relations activities. Healthcare organizations are typically regulated by organizations within their state and, for some purposes, by federal agencies. The reimbursement available to healthcare providers may be controlled by the appropriate regulatory agencies, and not-for-profit organizations must continuously demonstrate to government agencies that they deserve their tax-exempt status. For these reasons, healthcare organizations must maintain discourse with a variety of government agencies, cultivate relationships with politicians and other policy makers, and often initiate lobbying activities directed toward various levels of government. While some level of communication with government agencies may occur through the regular submission of reports, meaningful communication typically requires personal contact. Thus, the government relations staff of a large hospital, for example, would spend considerable time meeting with officials representing various governmental or regulatory entities.

Networking

Networking involves developing and nurturing relationships with individuals and organizations with which mutually beneficial transactions might be carried out. Physicians and other clinicians who, until recently, would never deign to advertise, actively network among their colleagues. This may involve a specialist casually running into potential referring physicians at the country club or attending meetings that might involve potential clients, partners or referral agents. Arranging activities (e.g., golf tournaments) that would bring together various parties with whom one might want to interact would be another form of networking. Networking is particularly effective when dealing with parties with whom it is hard to get "face time" or when one desires an informal setting involving personal interaction for getting to know prospective business associates.

While some formal networking activities may be used to communicate with selected audiences, much of the networking that takes place in healthcare is informal in nature. The communication that underlies the establishment and maintenance of referral relationships among healthcare providers is a prime example of this.

Sales Promotion

"Sales promotion" involves an activity or material that acts as a direct inducement to consumers by offering added value to a product or
incentives for resellers, salespersons or consumers. Sales promotions (e.g.,
rebates) are more likely to be associated with the sale of consumer health
products or business-to-business healthcare sales (e.g., low-interest financing) than with the provision of health services. The sales promotion mix
could, however, include fairs and trade shows, exhibits, demonstrations,
contests and games, premiums and gifts, rebates, low-interest financing,
and/or trade-in allowances. Sales promotion is separate from, but often
adjunct to, personal sales.

Sales promotion is typically associated with for-profit healthcare organizations. However, as competition has intensified in healthcare, both
for-profit and not-for-profit organizations have begun to utilize some of the
techniques usually associated with consumer industries. Certainly public
venues such as health fairs and expos are frequented by healthcare organizations at which they often distribute gifts, favors and other "promotional"
materials.

Advertising

"Advertising" refers to any paid form of non-personal presentation
and promotion of ideas, goods or services by an identifiable sponsor transmitted via mass media for purposes of achieving marketing objectives.
The advertising mix could include print advertising, electronic advertising, mailings, catalogues, brochures, posters, directories, outdoor ads
and displays. These activities are organized in the form of an advertising
"campaign" that involves designing a series of advertisements and placing them in various advertising media to reach a particular target market.
Healthcare organizations may even use innovative advertising vehicles
to reach their audiences, such as a weight loss program running an advertisement in a movie theatre or an HIV/AIDS program utilizing public
restroom advertising.

Advertising in print media has long been utilized by healthcare organizations. The primary venue is the daily newspaper, although weeklies,
alternative newspapers, and even "shoppers" may be utilized. Magazines
may also serve as a venue for advertising, although their less frequent
publication may make them less attractive.

Electronic media have come to dominate the advertising field, initially
with radio and then television capturing the imagination of "ad-men". The
use of these media has ebbed and flowed in healthcare, reflecting whatever the current thinking is with regard to health services marketing. These
media obviously have a lot of advantages for information dissemination,

although they have some drawbacks in terms of costs and questionable effectiveness. The emergence of social marketing in healthcare has resulted in a newfound interest in advertising. (See Box 9.2 for insights into developing television advertisements.)

Box 9.2

Developing Effective Television Ads

The following "rules of thumb" apply when developing television advertisements.

General Guidelines

- Keep messages short and simple—just one or two key points.
- Use language and style appropriate for the intended audience.
- Repeat the main message as many times as possible.
- Recommend a specific action.
- Demonstrate the health problem, behavior, or skill (if relevant).
- Provide new, accurate, straightforward information.
- Be sure the message, language, and style are considered relevant by the intended audience.
- Be sure that the message presenter is seen as a credible source of information, whether an authority, celebrity, or intended audience representative.

Development Approach

- Select an appropriate approach (e.g., testimonial, demonstration, or slice-of-life format).
- Be sure every word works.
- Use a memorable slogan, theme, music, or sound effects to aid recall.
- Check for consistency with campaign messages in other media formats.

Type of Appeal

- Use positive rather than negative appeals.
- Emphasize the solution as well as the problem.
- Use a light, humorous approach, if appropriate, but pretest to be sure that it works and doesn't offend the intended audience.
- Avoid high degrees of fear arousal, unless the fear is easily resolved and the message is carefully tested.

Box 9.2 (Continued).

Use of Visuals

- Use only a few characters.
- Make the message understandable from the visual portrayal alone.
- Superimpose text on the screen to reinforce the oral message's main point.

Timing Considerations

- Identify the main issue in the first 10 seconds in an attention-getting way.
- Use 30-second spots to present and repeat the complete message; use 10-second spots only for reminders.
- If the action is to call, show the phone number on the screen for at least 5 seconds, and reinforce orally.
- Summarize or repeat the main point/message at the close.

Source: National Cancer Institute (2003). *Making health communication work*. Washington: U.S. Government Printing Office.

Personal Sales

"Personal sales" involves the oral presentation of promotional material in a conversation with one or more prospective purchasers for the purpose of making sales. The process attempts to achieve mutually profitable economic exchanges between buyer and seller, based on interpersonal contact and the seller's persuasive communication of his product or service's qualities and its benefits for the buyer. The personal selling mix could include sales presentations, sales meetings, incentive programs, distribution of samples, and fairs and trade shows. Personal sales in healthcare are generally utilized for purposes of business-to-business promotions, although they may be used by fund-raisers in healthcare to solicit contributions from major donors.

Direct Mail

Although healthcare organizations were slow to adopt some of the more targeted approaches to consumer solicitation, some healthcare organizations have utilized direct mail as a form of communication. This approach involves the mailing of promotional materials to households in specified geographical areas or households with certain characteristics. This represents a more targeted form of communication than most other approaches and is discussed further in the next chapter. The attributes of direct mail include the identification of high potential consumers, the tailoring of the message to appeal to these consumers, and delivery of the message directly to their homes. Direct mail campaigns generally include some type of "call to action" whereby the recipient can take appropriate action if desired.

Direct mail can be an expensive proposition and generates relatively low yields. (Marketers in consumer industries typically have to accept a two percent response rate.) Further, households receive so much "junk mail" that, unless the mailer stands out in some way, it may not even be read. The only possible advantage for health communicators is that people seem more likely to look at material that appears to have come from a medical facility or healthcare organization.

Social Marketing

Social marketing is defined as "the application of commercial marketing technologies to the analysis, planning, execution, and evaluation of programs designed to influence the voluntary behavior of target audiences in order to improve their personal welfare and that of their society" (Andreason, 1995). Characteristics of the social marketing approach include:

1. A focus on benefits for targeted individuals and not on profit and organizational benefits;
2. A focus on behavior, not awareness or attitude change;
3. An approach that encourages the target audience's participation.

Social marketing has become increasingly common in healthcare as communicators have sought more effective means of reaching their audiences. Social marketing should not be considered a unitary method since it represents a multi-faceted, integrated approach to communicating health information. According to Weinreich (1999), social marketing has evolved from a one-dimensional reliance on public service announcements to a more sophisticated approach which draws from successful techniques used by commercial marketers. Rather than dictating the way that information is to be conveyed from the top-down, health professionals are learning to listen to the needs and desires of the target audience, and building the program accordingly. This focus on the "consumer" involves in-depth research and constant re-evaluation of every aspect of the program.

Social marketing has been used extensively in international health programs, especially for contraceptives and oral rehydration therapy (ORT), and is being used with more frequency in the United States for addressing such diverse topics as drug abuse, heart disease and organ donation.

Like commercial marketing, the primary focus is on learning what people want and need rather than trying to persuade them to buy what the organization is selling. Social marketing talks to the consumer, not about the product.

In social marketing, the formulation of the four Ps of the marketing mix (price, product, promotion, and place) is based upon research on consumers to identify acceptable benefits and costs and determine how they might best be reached. Lessons learned from social marketing stress the importance of understanding the intended audiences and designing strategies based on their wants and needs rather than what good health practice dictates.

Spokespersons

Many healthcare organizations utilize spokespersons of one type or another to gain visibility or credibility for their services. Spokespersons are thought to have many of the traits that make for effective communication—recognition, credibility, authority, and so forth. Spokespersons can take a variety of forms, depending on the nature of the organization, the material being presented, and the ultimate goal of the communication initiative. These may include individuals who have had experience with the service or have an interest in promoting a particular idea or behavior. In some cases, celebrity spokespersons may be hired to communicate a message although they have no other experience with or ties to the organization involved in communication.

Testimonials presented by individuals who have been served by the organization appear to be effective—the rehabilitation patient who has regained his capabilities, the former smoker from the smoking cessation program, the heart attack survivor. If these individuals happen to be well known locally or nationally, so much the better. A successful childbirth by a well-known actress at the facility or the successful rehabilitation of a star athlete would be welcomed by any health communicator.

Not all individuals, whether the man off the street or the national celebrity, make good spokespersons. Care should be taken to assure that the spokesperson chosen has the traits necessary for effective communication and presents the type of image that the organization wants to project. Plenty of examples can be cited of celebrity spokespersons who were expeditiously dropped because of something they said or did unrelated to the material being communicated.

MAXIMIZING MEDIA COVERAGE

Regardless of which approach it utilized, it is important to maximize media coverage. The following rules can be applied to this end:

- Know what different publications, stations, and shows typically cover, and which staff, editors, and reporters are responsible for what.
- Understand the media market in terms of what various members of the media see as their respective roles.
- Respond quickly to requests for information.
- Provide information the media can use.
- Be honest about your issue, your organization, what you know, what you can do for the media, and what you want from them.
- Work personally with the media to help them understand your issue.
- Ask for something the media can give besides coverage.
- Produce variations of materials to appeal to specific intended audience segments.
- Get the intended audience's attention.
- Produce high quality materials.
- Entertain while you educate when using mass media.

It is important to be sensitive to the needs and expectations of the media. Box 9.3 presents some of the likes and dislikes of the media.

Box 9.3

What Do the Media Like and Not Like?

Experience indicates that the media can be utilized most effectively if the health communicator is aware of what representatives of the various media like and don't like. Some of the key points in this regard are presented below:

What Do the Media Like?

- Stories with audience appeal
- Issues that stimulate debate, controversy, or conflict
- Stories that create higher ratings and larger audiences
- Fresh angles or twists on issues that will attract public interest
- Accurate background information
- Articles related to current or timely issues
- Human interest angles

Box 9.3 (Continued).

What Do the Media Dislike?

- Covering old topics
- Duplicating stories reported by competitors
- A lot of statistics
- Inaccuracies or incomplete content
- Articles on highly complex issues
- Receiving numerous calls when on a deadline
- People who persist when a story idea is rejected

COMBINATION OR INTEGRATED COMMUNICATION

A one-dimensional approach to the promotion of a health issue, such as reliance on mass media campaigns or other single-component communication activities, has been shown to be insufficient to achieve program goals. Successful health promotion efforts increasingly rely on multidimensional interventions to reach diverse audiences about complex health concerns, with communication integrated from the beginning with other components, such as community-based programs, policy changes, and improvements in services and the health delivery system. Research shows that health communication is most effective when multiple communication channels are used to reach specific audience segments with information that is appropriate and relevant to them.

During the design of multidimensional programs it is important to allot sufficient time for planning, implementation, and evaluation and sufficient money to support the many elements of the program. Public-private partnerships and collaborations can leverage resources to strengthen the impact of multidimensional efforts. Collaboration can have the added benefit of reducing message clutter and targeting health concerns that cannot be fully addressed by public resources or market incentives alone.

Using several different channels increases the likelihood of reaching more of the intended audiences. It also can increase repetition of the message, improving the chance that intended audiences will be exposed to it often enough to absorb and act upon it. For these reasons, a combination of channels has been found most effective in producing desired results, including behavior change (Center for Substance Abuse Prevention, 1996).

For example, Center for Substance Abuse Prevention (CSAP) communication grantees have combined channels in unique ways that reflect their communities. One grantee used posters in community facilities, placed radio spots, and distributed brochures through community sites and requests by radio listeners. Another used a satellite network to show videos, made small group presentations through organizations, and worked with schools to promote at-home activities. Yet another promoted its message through a music and visual arts training program that resulted in a live performance and television broadcast of the program's art and musical creations.

References

Andreason, A. (1995). *Marketing social change: Changing behavior to promote health, social development, and the environment.* San Francisco: Jossey-Bass.

Center for Substance Abuse Prevention Communications Cooperative Agreements. (1996). *Bridging the gap for people with disabilities.* Rockville, MD: US Department of Health and Human Services.

Weinreich, Nedra Kline (1999). *Hands-on social marketing : A step-by-step guide.* Thousand Oaks, CA: Sage.

Additional Resources

Centers for Disease Control and Prevention. (1996). *The prevention marketing initiative: Applying prevention marketing* (CDC Publication No. D905). Atlanta.

Centers for Disease Control and Prevention. (2000). *Beyond the brochure* (CDC Publication No. PDF-821K). Atlanta.

Kotler, P., & Roberto, E. L. (1989). *Social marketing: Strategies for changing public behavior.* New York: Free Press.

Lefebvre, R. C., & Rochlin, L. (1997). Social marketing. In K. Glanz, F. M. Lewis, & B. K. Rimer (Eds.), *Health behavior and health education: Theory, research, and practice* (2nd ed.). San Francisco: Jossey-Bass.

Chapter 10

Contemporary Approaches to Health Communication

C hapter 10 reviews contemporary approaches to health communication, including those that incorporate state-of-the-art technology capabilities. Communication as a field has experienced a number of changes in recent years and these developments have affected healthcare. Emerging techniques from direct-to-consumer initiatives to e-marketing campaigns are discussed. The role of electronic information distribution is discussed, along with the advantages and disadvantages of technology-based communication.

FACTORS CONTRIBUTING TO EMERGING TECHNIQUES

The 1990s witnessed the adoption of techniques from other industries and the development of new healthcare-specific approaches to communication. Numerous developments in healthcare over the past two decades have led to a need for innovative communication techniques. The significance of customer relationship management, direct-to-consumer marketing and other emerging techniques cannot be overlooked. The shift from an emphasis on communicating with the "masses" to one on communication with specific segments of the market has led to new and different approaches to communication.

Developments in the communication field reflect a number of trends related to healthcare. These include a shift in emphasis from image marketing to service marketing and movement away from a mass marketing approach to a more targeted approach. As a result, healthcare communication

133

has experienced a move away from a one-size-fits-all philosophy to one that emphasizes personalization and customization. There has also been a shift away from an emphasis on the specific healthcare episode to an emphasis on long-term relationships.

A number of factors have contributed to the changing character of health communication and, in the new millennium, the field promises to be quite different from that of the last century. There are factors that are pushing the field in a new direction and others that are pulling it. The most important factors in this regard are described below.

Push Factors

The following factors in recent years have served to encourage new approaches to communication in healthcare.

Consumerism.   Toward the end of the twentieth century, the consumer was "rediscovered" by the American healthcare industry. The consumer—the ultimate end-user of health services and products—had long been written off as a marketing target. For most medical services, the physician made the decisions for the patient and, for the insured, the health plan controlled the choice of provider and the range of services that could be obtained from that provider. The choice of drug typically depended on the physician's prescription, and supply channels in general focused on the "middle man" rather than the end-user (Thomas, 2004).

The rise of the baby boomers into dominance within the U.S. population contributed greatly to the consumer movement in healthcare. Boomers were more educated and expected more options from life. Higher incomes supported the lifestyles to which they quickly became accustomed. With the oldest boomers turning 55 at the beginning of the twenty-first century, the healthcare system will soon experience the onslaught of the aging boomer. Boomers, however, are not going to accept their aging fate without a fight. Their youth taught them the power of consumerism, their college years taught them the power of a collective voice, and their careers taught them the power of money. It is these lessons, combined with their overall skepticism of the healthcare institution, that are going to restructure healthcare as we know it.

Growing Market Orientation.   By the 1980s healthcare had become increasingly market driven. Healthcare providers needed to know what the patient liked and did not like about the services provided. Marketers were called upon to not only identify the wants and needs of the market, but to assist in maintaining a high level of customer satisfaction. The rise of consumerism and growing competition meant that the market was now driving the bus. This invariably resulted in stepped-up communication with the consumers who constituted the market.

Health Disparities. The existence of health disparities among different groups in U.S. society is a longstanding problem. Members of various racial and ethnic groups, inner city residents, and the economically disadvantaged are among the groups that suffer disparities in health status, access to care, and treatment by the healthcare system. The fact that the disparities appear to be growing rather than declining suggests that current remedial efforts are not very effective. Part of the blame must be attributed to the ineffectiveness of health communication, since it is clear that gaps remain in the healthcare knowledge of many subgroups in the population and in their ability to utilize the system.

The Need for Social Marketing. Public sector organizations have been faced with a need to get their message to the consumer but with limited means to do so. The concept of social marketing emerged as public health agencies developed campaigns to inform the public of the dangers of smoking and drinking, methods of reducing the spread of sexually transmitted diseases, and the importance of prenatal care. Formal marketing techniques provided a channel for disseminating information that had not been successfully transmitted in a wholesale fashion in the past.

Information Requirements. As healthcare became more complex and healthcare organizations offered a growing array of services, the demand for information on the part of customers and the general public alike increased. Information and referral requirements called for more effective approaches to data management and information dissemination. This forced health professionals to turn to more sophisticated technical solutions for generating, processing and disseminating information.

Population-based Approach. A growing body of research indicates that the traditional one-on-one approach used to address health problems has not been effective in improving the health status of the U.S. population. The situation calls for more of a population-based approach through which large groups within the population can be influenced. This requires a different communication approach than those historically utilized and increases the applications of social marketing.

Pull Factors

The following factors have encouraged movement toward more contemporary forms of communication.

Data Management Capabilities. Dramatic strides have been made in data management capabilities in recent years and health professionals, although lagging behind those in other industries, are beginning to take advantage of the potential. Cognizant of HIPAA restrictions, healthcare organizations have developed increasingly sophisticated means of capturing, processing, managing and exploiting consumer data. These capabilities provide the foundation for many of the more contemporary forms of communication.

Developments in Telecommunication. Led by the Internet, improvements in telecommunication capabilities are transforming the healthcare field. The opportunities for communicating health information have increased dramatically and the Internet is rapidly becoming not only the primary source of health-related information but the conduit for much data transfer and the venue for interaction between patients, providers and other players in the industry. After stalling for many years, telemedicine is beginning to become established as an important component of the healthcare system.

Developments in Marketing. The foundation of marketing is effective communication and the healthcare marketing field has matured dramatically over the past couple of decades. As marketing overall has become more sophisticated, many of these capabilities have been adopted by healthcare. Health communication is in a position to take advantage of these developments and adapt them for use in healthcare.

THE REORIENTATION OF COMMUNICATION

The shift toward more contemporary approaches to health communication has been driven by a number of developments in society and healthcare. The most important of these developments are discussed below.

From Episode to Relationship

There has been a shift away from an emphasis on the specific healthcare episode to an emphasis on long-term relationships. Until recently, the intent of health communication was to convey a set body of information, bring about a specific action, or otherwise address a problem in a relatively restricted manner. While prevention has always been a target of communication, the contemporary approach takes even a longer-range view and addresses individuals from before they are at risk to long after the clinical episode has taken place. The communication approach required to maintain a long-term relationship differs from that required to affect an episode.

From Knowledge Transfer to Behavior Change

Similar to the previous point, communication in healthcare appears to be moving from an emphasis on knowledge transfer to one on behavior change. Research has found that information by itself may not overcome attitudes, perceptions, lack of motivation and other barriers to health-seeking behavior. Effective communication must motivate individuals to change their behaviors and provide the support necessary for them to overcome the many barriers to effective management of their health.

From Macro to Micro

Like marketing in general, health communication has historically taken a mass marketing approach to the dissemination of information. Not so much that health communicators used the mass media, but that they packaged materials to appeal to the broadest possible audience. This one-size-fits-all approach has become increasingly ineffective over time and, like the marketing industry, health communication has moved first to target marketing and then to micro-marketing in an attempt to reach specific audiences.

"Target marketing" refers to marketing initiatives that focus on a market segment to which an organization desires to offer goods or services. While mass marketing involves a shotgun approach, target marketing is more of a rifle approach. Target markets in healthcare may be defined based on geography, demographics, lifestyles, insurance coverage, usage rates and/or other customer attributes.

"Micromarketing" is a form of target marketing in which marketers tailor their marketing programs to the needs and wants of narrowly defined geographic, demographic, psychographic, or benefit segments. Customers and potential customers are identified at the household or individual level in order to promote goods and/or services directly to selected targets. Micromarketing is most effective when consumers with a narrow range of attributes must be reached. The ability to take a "mass customization" approach has changed the nature of health communication.

From Individual Focus to Population Focus

A trend seemingly in contrast to the previous one is the shift in emphasis from the individual to the population as a target for information dissemination and health intervention. Community-centered prevention shifts attention from the individual to group-level change and emphasizes the empowerment of individuals and communities to effect change on multiple levels. A growing appreciation for the contextual and environmental influences on health status and health behavior and a concern for the overall well-being of the population has prompted an interest in approaches to health problems (and, by extension, health communication) that hopes to affect the condition of groups of people rather than separate individuals. While this may seem counter to the shift from a macro to a micro communication approach, the ability to mass customize messages makes it possible to address consumers in both manners.

EMERGING COMMUNICATION TECHNIQUES

The emerging approaches to health communication can be thought to have three common characteristics: 1) use of technology; 2) adoption from other industries; and 3) the establishment of relationships. Increasingly, health communication professionals are taking advantage of digital technologies, such as CD-ROM and the World Wide Web, that can target audiences, tailor messages, and engage people in interactive, ongoing exchanges about health. Health professionals have also come to recognize both the value of more formal marketing techniques and the lessons that can be learned from other industries. Rather than "reinventing the wheel", health communicators have the opportunity to benefit from developments in communication techniques in other fields.

Relationship development focuses on the establishment of long-term relationships through careful attention to customer needs and service delivery. Relationship marketing is characterized by: 1) a focus on customer retention, 2) an orientation towards product benefits rather than product features, 3) a long-term view of the relationship, 4) maximum emphasis on customer commitment and contact, 5) development of on-going relationship, 6) multiple employee/customer contacts, 7) an emphasis on key account relationship management, 8) and an emphasis on trust. All of the techniques discussed below incorporate at least some of these attributes.

The communication techniques that appear to be gaining momentum in healthcare can perhaps be divided into techniques that involve organizational changes and those that are technology based. The former implies an innovative approach at a conceptual level and the latter a technology-based approach as applied to either traditional or innovative communication techniques.

Organizational Approaches

Direct-to-Consumer Approaches

The direct-to-consumer (DTC) movement is gaining momentum in healthcare as the industry becomes more consumer driven and the ability to target narrow population segments becomes more refined. Healthcare marketers are modifying their methodologies to take into consideration the potential represented by 280 million prospective customers. This involves a radical rethinking of traditional approaches to healthcare audiences.

In many ways, DTC marketing is the offspring of the direct marketing activities of previous years. "Direct marketing" is a form of marketing that targets specific groups or individuals with specific characteristics and subsequently transmits promotional messages directly to them. These promotional activities may take the form of direct mail or telemarketing, as well as other approaches aimed at specific individuals. Increasingly, the Internet is being utilized for direct marketing. An advantage of direct marketing is that the message can be customized to meet the needs of narrowly defined target populations.

With the rediscovery of the healthcare consumer, all of this is undergoing dramatic change. Aided by access to state-of-the-art technology, consumers are now expressing their preferences for everything from physicians and hospitals to health plans to prescription drugs. And now, direct-to-consumer advertising is beginning to emerge as a force in healthcare.

The DTC movement has been given a jump start by the pharmaceutical industry. Once certain restrictions to DTC advertising were removed, the pharmaceutical giants began targeting the consumer through a variety of media. This industry is currently leading the way in terms of expenditures and visibility as pharmaceutical interests attempt to attract consumers to their brands.

This trend has been followed, albeit at a safe distance, by various health insurance plans that are beginning to offer their policies via the Internet—thereby causing a resurgence in insurance plans aimed at individuals rather than groups. The accelerating shift from defined benefits to defined contributions is rapidly making the ability to customize health plans to the needs of specific groups—and, indeed, individuals—essential for any health plan that hopes to remain competitive.

The reemergence of the consumer has not been lost on practitioners either, as hospitals, physicians, and other providers establish Web sites for maintaining contact with existing customers and enticing prospective customers. Now it is possible to bid on an elective procedure (a facelift by a plastic surgeon, for example), thereby establishing a direct negotiating link between provider and consumer. Direct mail is also experiencing a resurgence among providers, as the importance of DTC marketing becomes more apparent.

For their part, consumers have eagerly accepted this onslaught of direct marketing attention. Spearheaded by the baby boomers, a better educated, more affluent, and more control-oriented consumer population is eagerly searching for information tailored to their particular needs.

Much of the traffic on the Internet is health oriented, and today's consumers obtain much of their health-related information via the World Wide Web.

Although the Internet has served to give impetus to much of the new attention targeted directly to individual consumers, the DTC movement has affected other media as well. In addition to the Internet, television and print media have experienced a considerable increase in expenditures. While much of this has been driven by the pharmaceutical industry, there is no reason to expect that other parties chasing these same consumers will not follow suit.

The need to target large numbers of consumers has triggered a surge of interest in psychographics and other consumer profiling methodologies. In the past, if you knew a couple of things about a patient or potential patient (e.g., referring doctor, health plan), you did not need to know much more. In the future, the ability to contact and subsequently cultivate prospective patients is going to place significant pressure on the marketer.

Business-to-Business Communication

Although much of the discussion around health communication focuses on the patient or other end-user, a significant amount of communication in healthcare involves business-to-business transactions. The increasing corporatization of healthcare means that more and more relationships are between one corporate body and another. The traditional doctor-patient relationship has been supplanted by contractual arrangements between groups of buyers and sellers of health services. Many hospital programs now target corporate customers rather than individual patients. The shift to a more business-like approach to healthcare delivery has also contributed to the growth of business-to-business marketing. From traditional public relations activities to contemporary technology-based approaches, the business customer is being given more emphasis.

Clearly, business-to-business communication in healthcare is nothing new. Healthcare organizations are major purchasers of a wide variety of goods, and large healthcare organizations do business with hundreds of vendors, but its importance is expected to increase in the future. Business-to-business marketing involves building profitable, value-oriented relationships between two businesses and the many individuals within them. Business marketers focus on a few customers, with usually much larger, more complex and technically oriented sales processes. Statistical tools, data mining techniques, and other sorts of research that work so well in the realm of consumer marketing must be fine-tuned and specially applied in the practice of the business marketer.

Business-to-business marketing is a complex discipline that has become integral to selling goods and services to business, industrial, institutional, or government buyers. In past decades, innovative products, great engineering, or great salesmanship alone might have been enough to close a business sale, but sellers no longer have the luxury of "build it and they will come" thinking. Business customers and traditional customers do not buy in the same way; they are driven by different impulses and respond to different types of appeals. As a consequences they require a different communication approach.

Technology-Based Approaches

Telemarketing

"Telemarketing" is a mechanism for directly communicating with consumers and one that most people are familiar with. It is not a new form of communication but is included in this chapter because of the use of contemporary technology. Most people are more familiar with outbound telemarketing in which individuals operating from a bank of telephone sets, often equipped with computer-assisted interviewing software, call individuals from a prospect list in order to offer a good or service.

Some telemarketing involves "cold calls" to individuals or households for which the demand for goods and services is unknown. More likely, the telephone numbers that are used as a sampling frame or are randomly generated relate to areas that have the approximate characteristics of the target audience. Inbound telemarketing involves processing incoming calls from individuals responding to some type of call-to-action that has been initiated.

A more benign form of telemarketing in healthcare involves periodic contacts with individuals who have expressed an interest to the healthcare organization with regard to a particular program or topic. It is assumed that the individual is willing to receive calls describing such programs and will not consider them an imposition due to their implied previous interest. Hospital call centers frequently use this approach to contact prospects for various services and programs.

Telemarketing is more expensive than direct mail initiatives, but the costs are not unreasonable. Wages for telemarketers are relatively low, and the benefits to a healthcare organization that attracts a new patient are likely to be significant. Obviously, not all healthcare products lend themselves to this approach but a surprising number do. Ultimately, telemarketing can represent a form of communication that, despite its negative image, can serve to build relationships with customers.

Database Marketing and CRM

"Database marketing" involves the establishment and exploitation of data on past and current customers together with future prospects, structured to allow for the implementation of effective communication strategies. Database marketing can be used for any purpose that can benefit from access to customer information. These functions may include evaluating new prospects, cross-selling related products, launching new products to potential prospects, identifying new distribution channels, building customer loyalty, converting occasional users into regular users, generating inquiries and follow-up sales, and establishing niche marketing initiatives. The database that is established for this purpose often provides the basis for customer relationship management (CRM) and may be an integral part of an organization's call center.

"Customer relationship management" (CRM) is a business strategy designed to optimize profitability, revenue and customer satisfaction by focusing on customer relationships rather than transactions. This has become an inevitable outgrowth of the emergence of database marketing. While long utilized in other industries, CRM is relatively new to healthcare. The industry's lack of focus on customer characteristics and limited data management capabilities have retarded the acceptance of CRM in healthcare. However, the new, market-driven environment is encouraging the development of customer databases and their use by healthcare organizations.

Increasingly, health improvement activities are taking advantage of digital technologies, such as CD-ROM and the World Wide Web, that can target audiences, tailor messages, and engage people in interactive, ongoing exchanges about health. As population-based approaches to healthcare have become more common, the role of health communication has expanded. Community-centered prevention shifts attention from the individual to group-level change and emphasizes the empowerment of individuals and communities to effect change on multiple levels.

Interactive Health Communication

"Interactive health communication" (IHC) can be defined as the interaction of an individual—consumer, patient, caregiver, or professional—with an electronic device or communication technology to access or transmit health information or to receive guidance on a health-related issue. Examples of IHC include Websites devoted to health and/or healthcare, online chat groups, listservs and news groups, stand-alone information kiosks, and CD-ROM applications. These vehicles for IHC perform the functions of relaying information, enabling informed decision making, promoting healthy behavior, promoting peer information exchange and support, promoting self-care, and managing the demand for health services (Science Panel on Interactive Communications, 1999).

Advances in medical and consumer health informatics are changing the delivery of health information and services and are likely to have a growing impact on individual and community health. The convergence of media (computers, telephones, television, radio, video, print, and audio) and the emergence of the Internet create a nearly ubiquitous networked communication infrastructure. This infrastructure facilitates access to an increasing array of health information and health-related support services and extends the reach of health communication efforts. Delivery channels such as the Internet expand the choices available for health professionals to reach patients and consumers and for patients and consumers to interact with health professionals and with each other (for example, in online support groups).

Compared to traditional mass media, interactive media have several advantages when it comes to health communication. These advantages include (1) improved access to personalized health information, (2) access to health information, support, and services on demand, (3) enhanced ability to distribute materials widely and update content or functions rapidly, (4) just-in-time expert decision support, and (5) more choices for consumers.

Although healthcare organizations were slow to jump on the Internet bandwagon, recent years have seen a surge of interest in the use of the Internet for a wide range of communication initiatives in healthcare. Most hospitals have Websites up and running, and some healthcare organizations have actually led the way with regard to some aspects of on-line communication.

Significant growth has occurred in the number of consumers who search for healthcare information online. Whether it is a patient or a caregiver, the Internet is used as a resource both before and after visiting the doctor. Because these are information seekers, they are receptive to information provided healthcare organizations. Some of the aura surrounding the Internet has been diminished due to the bad experience with dot.coms. Yet, there continues to be growth in the public interest in online healthcare information and evidence that increasingly numbers of healthcare consumers are logging on. (The importance of an effective Web presence cannot be overlooked and Box 10.1 describes some of the features of an effective Website.)

Healthcare Websites generally have moved the beyond static marketing information and corporate descriptions, introducing a deeper level of

Box 10.1

Developing and Promoting an Effective Website

Based on its research on effective Websites for health communication, the National Cancer Institute (2003) identified a number of "rules" for successful sites. To ensure that users will find the site well designed and easy to use, the site should be pretested just like any other materials. Usability testing, which tests the site to see how well it helps users meet their goals, is crucial to creating an effective site. The best time to do this testing is during development, not after it's completed. If the site is not yet running on a computer, it should be tested using paper or poster board mock-ups of pages. Usability testing can be conducted by having people who represent the intended audience use the site to complete tasks. Interaction with the site can be observed and specific questions asked once they have completed the tasks. Their experiences and responses will allow for prerelease modifications. If major modifications are made to the site after usability testing, the site should be tested again before it goes live. (For more information on usability testing, see www.usability.gov.)

A well-designed and attractive site is useless unless people know it exists. Therefore, both traditional and online media approaches should be considered during the launch. Online outreach can include alerting search engines such as Google or Yahoo about the site, as well as selecting publications that specialize in online issues.

According to the National Cancer Institute, an effective Website should have the following attributes:
- Compliant with W3C accessibility guidelines
- Clean and consistent design
- A search engine and a link to the search engine on all Web pages
- Rapid display of graphics and text
- Clear and consistent navigation functions

A Website should be graphically appealing and provide information about health issues in an informative manner. Some organizations begin by creating sites that primarily provide information to their stakeholders, employees, or members. To extend outreach, an additional section might be created in the site to appeal to the intended audience. Many sites contain useful public health information and resources, but too often this information is buried within the site.

Source: National Cancer Institute (2003). *Making health communication work*. Washington: U.S. Government Printing Office.

service line and health content and more interactive features and applications. Most are still far from being truly integrated with the marketing efforts or other information technology applications of their organization. An increasing number of health systems are pushing customized health information and medical records out to consumers, allowing e-mail communication with physicians and doing some level of actual disease management online.

The Internet offers more than just a source of one-way information transfer. It is increasingly becoming a primary means of conducting healthcare transactions. These might include completing a health risk appraisal online, scheduling a physician appointment, ordering a healthcare product, or interacting with a caregiver. Healthcare providers are increasingly using the Internet to "push" information out to consumers and monitor the activities of their clients. Offering health plan sign-up, status and benefit changes online at a worksite kiosk or home computer adds "place" value. The ability to have one's medical record available on line has added a different dimension to the concept of place.

Many healthcare organizations and public service agencies use the Internet as one of their main channels for information delivery. Access to the Internet and subsequent technologies is likely to become essential to gain access to health information, contact healthcare organizations and health professionals, receive services at a distance, and participate in efforts to improve local and national health. The integration of communication media means electronic access to health information not only via computers but also with Web-enabled televisions and telephones, handheld devices, and other emerging technologies. Technical literacy, or the ability to use electronic technologies and applications, will be essential to gain access to this information.

Internet availability in the home is an important indicator of equitable access among population groups. An increasing number of people have access to the Internet at work or at public facilities, such as libraries and community centers, but several limitations affect the use of online health information and support in these settings. Some employers monitor electronic mail and the types of sites visited by employees. Access in public settings may be problematic because of privacy and confidentiality concerns, and access may be needed during times when these facilities are unavailable. Because of the potentially sensitive nature of health-related uses of the Internet, access at home will ultimately be essential.

Although "internal marketing" in not generally thought of as a "contemporary" approach to health communication, its importance in the new healthcare environment cannot be overlooked. Box 10.2 describes some of the issues involved in internal marketing for health communicators.

Box 10.2

Fostering Internal Communication

Internal communication refers to efforts by a service provider to effectively train and motivate its customer-contact employees and all supporting service staff to work as a team to generate customer satisfaction. This does not represent a new and innovative technique so much as a shift in emphasis. Internal communication aims to ensure that everybody within an organization is working towards the achievement of common objectives. It recognizes that people who work together stand in exactly the same relationships to each other as do customers and suppliers. Internal marketing represents a marketing effort, inside a company's four walls, that targets internal audiences. Its goal is to increase communications among staff members so that a marketing campaign's effectiveness is maximized.

Internal communication redefines employees as valued customers. The rationale is that anticipating, identifying and satisfying employee needs will lead to greater commitment. This in turn will allow the organization to improve the quality of service to its external customers.

The communication department is a logical focal point for internal marketing due to its knowledge of the organization's overall strategy, its appreciation of external customer's needs, the expertise to deploy these tools with regard to internal customers, and the budgets and financial resources to do the job.

A primary goal of internal communication is to make employees fully aware of the aims and activities of the organization. It is amazing how often employees of large healthcare organizations are unaware of services or programs the organization offers. While this could happen in any organization, it appears to be an inherent characteristic of healthcare organizations. Employees must also be given a basic understanding of the nature of the customer. Employees of healthcare organizations are often isolated from the service delivery aspects of the operation. They may have virtually no knowledge of the customer interaction process or at best a partial understanding of service delivery.

Lack of investment in internal communication may be the result of corporate distraction. Companies that are frantically trying to boost revenues and cut costs may not see why they should spend money on employees—missing the point that these are the very people who ultimately deliver the brand promises the company makes.

Lack of investment may also reflect a conscious decision by executives who dismiss internal efforts as feel-good pseudo-science—missing

Box 10.2 (Continued).

the point that research consistently demonstrates that service quality problems (people problems more than product problems) are what push customers away and into the arms of competitors.

Internal communication is also an important implementation tool. It facilitates information transfer and helps overcome resistance to change. It is simple to construct especially if traditional principles of marketing are applied. Internal marketing obeys the same rules as, and has a similar structure to, external marketing. The main differences are that the customers are staff and colleagues from the organization.

Among the most common features of internal communication efforts are meetings, special events, company anniversary celebrations, appreciation dinners, brown bag lunches, off-site/satellite offices visits, internal newsletters, bulletin boards, e-mail newsletters, intranets, and broadcast e-mails.

References

Science Panel on Interactive Communication and Health. (1999). *Wired for health and well-being: The emergence of interactive health communication.* Washington, DC: US Department of Health and Human Services, US Government Printing Office.

Thomas, Richard K. (2004). *Marketing health services.* Chicago, IL: Health Administration Press.

Chapter 11

Case Studies in Health Communication

C hapter 11 presents a number of case studies that reflect the application of varying techniques to different health communication audiences. Examples of traditional health communication approaches are
presented along with cases reflecting the application of contemporary technology. Campaigns designed to inform, motivate or change behavior are
described, with examples targeting individuals, organization and communities offered. An attempt has been made to represent each aspect of the
communication process through a case study.

A CASE STUDY IN HEALTH COMMUNICATION RESEARCH:
MEDIA PREFERENCES OF YOUNG WORKERS

A major national corporation became concerned about the problem of
substance abuse among its youthful employees. In order to effectively reach
this population, employee assistance personnel within the corporation felt
they needed to identify the types of media that might influence young
employees. Because of the geographic dispersion of their workforce, they
felt that a lifestyle segmentation approach would allow them to classify
their employees in terms of communication preferences. Using the Mosaic
lifestyle segmentation system developed by Experian, they first identified
the lifestyle segments into which the majority of their young workers fell.
They then identified the most common media channels through which
these employees received their information. The major lifestyle clusters
and their media preferences are listed below:

Cluster	Media Preferences
Second City Homebodies	Regular movie watching; cable TV; ethnic oriented radio/television; not big readers
Urban Optimists	Heavy ethnic-oriented radio; high movie attendance and light magazine readership; heavy into interactive Websites
Mid-market Enterprise	Heavy into Internet and other electronic media; not heavy readers
Southern Blues	Cable TV (black- and youth-oriented programming, movies); below average Internet usage
Urban Grit	Youngest of the clusters but well below average in PC/Internet use; urban contemporary and black-oriented radio; daytime television
Minority Metro Communities	Overwhelmingly black; average PC and Internet users; television for sports, information and entertainment; urban and new adult contemporary radio; black-oriented and religious radio; late night television; popular magazines and books

Information on the media preferences characteristic of the corporations' young workers provided the basis for developing communication initiatives that played to the interests of the target population.

A CASE STUDY IN HEALTH COMMUNICATION RESEARCH: DETERMINING CONSUMER PERCEPTIONS OF OBESITY

In an effort to determine the perceptions held by high-risk populations with regard to obesity and its causes and cures, four town hall meetings were held by a consortium of healthcare organizations in different communities in Memphis, Tennessee. Since the healthcare providers felt that they poorly understood perceptions of obesity within the community, the town hall meetings were intended to elicit feedback from low-income African Americans with regard to their ideas for addressing the issue. Although those providing input did not represent a scientifically drawn sample of residents of the targeted communities, they were thought to represent a reasonable cross-section of the target population.

The questions posed to the community residents in attendance were:

- What can family, friends and other associates do to help address the issue of obesity within the community?
- What can the community do to help address the issue of obesity among its residents?
- What can medical professionals do to help address the issue of obesity?

The recordings of the meeting proceedings were transcribed and conclusions were drawn with regard to participant knowledge about the obesity situation, participant attitudes toward obesity, factors contributing to the obesity "epidemic", and barriers to effectively addressing the problem. Some of the findings derived from the town hall meetings included:

- Participants have a reasonable knowledge of the problem of obesity, its causes and its associated dangers.
- Participants are generally aware of the importance of exercise and healthy dietary habits for good health.
- Participants generally accept the notion that there is no "quick fix" for an individual's obesity problem.
- Participants expressed a genuine concern about obesity for themselves and their families and a willingness to address the issue.
- Participants felt that obesity (and health in general) were issues that could be addressed if the necessary resources were available.
- Participants felt that there was a gap between the needs of the population and the health personnel and facilities available to meet them.
- While participants felt that most community residents were aware of the problem of obesity, they believed many did not have the knowledge, skills or resources necessary to effectively address the issue.
- While regular exercise was recognized as an important means of addressing obesity, participants contended that lack of access, prohibitive costs, and a lack of guidance with regard to exercise facilities were deterrents.
- Participants expressed concern that cultural factors within the community were deterrents to effectively addressing obesity.

The primary conclusion drawn from these meetings was: The ability of residents of the target communities to address obesity is not a function of a lack of knowledge or detrimental attitudes but a reflection of the lack of resources and an effective support structure to facilitate the changes that the residents know need to be made. The information gathered through these town hall meetings was used to design a grassroots communication initiative to address obesity within the disadvantaged African-American population.

A CASE STUDY IN CONCEPT TESTING

In 1996, the Office of Cancer Communications within the National Cancer Institute launched the Cancer Research Awareness Initiative to increase the public's understanding of medical research and the relevance of research breakthroughs for people's lives. The Office's efforts at concept development and message testing for this initiative were carried out in logical sequence. The following message concepts were developed and explored in focus groups with intended audience members:

- Research has led to real progress in the detection, diagnosis, treatment, and prevention of cancer.
- Everyone benefits from cancer research in some fashion.
- Cancer research is conducted in universities and medical schools across the country.
- Cancer research gives hope.
- At the broadest level, research priorities are determined by societal problems and concerns.
- At the project level, research priorities are driven primarily by past research successes and current opportunities.

Once feedback had been obtained from focus group participants concerning the importance of medical research of the target audience, the following messages were crafted:

1. Cancer Research: Discovering Answers for All of Us
2. Cancer Research: Because Cancer Touches Us All
3. Cancer Research: Discovering More Answers Every Day
4. Cancer Research: Because Lives Depend on It
5. Cancer Research: Only Research Cures Cancer

Once these messages had been developed, mall-intercept interviews were conducted to pretest them. Based on responses elicited from the intended audience in these interviews, message #4 was selected as the program theme.

A CASE STUDY IN PUBLIC SERVICE ANNOUNCEMENT DEVELOPMENT

Previous research has found that some youth have a preference for novel experiences and stimuli. In developing a communication campaign targeting youthful drug users, an approach that would appeal to young "sensation seekers" was designed. Sensation seekers fell into four subcategories representing different degrees of sensation seeking:

1. Thrill- and adventure-seeking (e.g., parachuting and scuba diving)
2. Experience-seeking (e.g., nonconforming lifestyle and musical tastes, drugs, unconventional friends)
3. Disinhibition (sensation through social stimulation; e.g., parties, social drinking, a variety of sex partners)
4. Boredom susceptibility (restlessness when things are the same for too long)

Health communicators working on drug abuse prevention programs endeavored to focus on sensation seekers with messages that appealed to this aspect of their personalities. The intent was to draw attention to the message and influence behavioral intentions and attitudes. To this end, University of Kentucky researchers designed a creative, high-sensation television public service announcement (PSA) that focused on the importance of alternatives to substance use for meeting sensation needs. The PSA, titled "Common," featured heavy metal music and quick-action cuts of high-sensation activities. "Wasted," which had the highest sensation value, also had heavy metal music and displayed the words "wasted," "blasted," "stoned," and "fried." Voice-over and illustrative footage accompanied each word (e.g., "with drugs you can get fried" had footage of a monk's self-immolation). It closed with the words "without drugs you can still get high" and offered examples of high-sensation alternatives.

Source: Palmgreen, P., et al. (1995). "Reaching at-risk populations in a mass media drug abuse prevention campaign: Sensation seeking as a targeting variable," in *Drugs & Society* 8(3), 29–45.

A CASE STUDY IN MESSAGE DEVELOPMENT

In order to provide cancer risk information to the public that could be readily understood and used, the National Cancer Institute (NCI) conducted a series of focus groups to learn what various groups thought of different methods for communicating about risks. The following insights from the research groups underscored the importance of considering both word usage and presentation methods when developing message concepts and materials:

- Participants said that they want cancer risk messages to give them hope for preventing cancer and that risk information is less threatening when written in optimistic terms.
- When faced with "bad news" about cancer risks, they said that they look for why it does not apply to them.
- They wanted risk messages to address key questions such as "How serious is the risk?" and "What can be done to reduce or avoid the risk?" as well as explain how and where to get additional information.
- Word choice also influences how information is perceived; "risk" raises alarm, while "chance" minimizes it.
- Use of vague or unfamiliar terms (including "fourfold," "relative risk," "lifetime risk") gives people reason to discount the information.
- Combining brief text and visuals (such as charts, graphs) can increase attention and understanding.
- Statistical risk information was difficult for many participants to understand; percentages were more understandable than ratios, but in either case accompanying explanations of the seriousness of the risk were needed.
- Participants were interested in "the complete picture"—that is, what is known and what is not yet known about a risk, and what it means for "human beings."

The source of risk information colors credibility, with participants saying that they are less likely to trust the media or a source with a business interest and more likely to trust risk information supplied by a physician or a medical journal.

Source: National Cancer Institute. (1998). *How the public perceives, processes, and interprets risk information: Findings from focus group research with the general public*. Washington, DC: U.S. Government Printing Office.

A CASE STUDY IN INCENTIVE DESIGN

In order to prevent the use of alcohol, tobacco and illicit drugs by youth, the Center for Substance Abuse Prevention within the U.S. Department of Health and Human Services partnered with the Girl Scouts of the U.S.A. to develop an incentive program. Built around the Girl Scout system for earning patches for completing specified assignments, the

Center assisted in the development of the Girl Power! program. The program involved a new patch to be awarded as an incentive for girls 9–14 to participate in the prevention program.

A national public health education program, Girl Power! addressed a wide range of issues affecting adolescent girls, with the overall goal of delaying and reducing the use of alcohol, tobacco, and illicit drugs. This program also addressed related issues such as physical activity, nutrition, and mental health. Through the Girl Scouts, the Center for Substance Abuse Prevention's Girl Power! materials were distributed to over 2.8 million girls around the country.

Under the auspice of the Center, the Girl Power! program was eventually expanded to cover a variety of health and lifestyle issues relevant to young girls. The centerpiece of the program is the Girl Power! website with sections for girls, grownups and researchers.

A CASE STUDY IN THE USE OF PEER COUNSELORS FOR TRANSMITTING AIDS INFORMATION

As the nature of the AIDS epidemic has changed, one of the growing challenges involves getting information in front of hard-to-reach populations. Among the fastest growing but hardest to reach subgroups suffering from HIV/AIDS is the African-American population. The AIDS Survival Project (ASP) in Georgia needed to reach the African-American community and help those living with HIV by providing a sympathetic ear and referrals to places that provide needed services.

One effective means of reaching this population developed by ASP involved the use of peer counselors. Peer counselors at the AIDS Survival Project take calls from persons living with or affected by HIV/AIDS. Callers and visitors include people who have family living with HIV, who are worried that they might have been exposed to HIV, or who want to know more about HIV and how it is transmitted. Peer counselors offer an added benefit to callers since they themselves are living with HIV, representing someone who has "been there, done that."

Those who volunteer as peer counselors are trained in how to find information for clients in the ASP Treatment Resource Center, on the Internet, or through the HIV resource database. Peer counselors also receive training in how to listen actively and interact with others in a non-judgmental manner. These skills facilitate peer counseling while helping the volunteers themselves cope more effectively with their condition.

Source: Smith, Jeff (2001). "Peer counseling perspectives," *Survival News* (September). Downloaded from URL: http://thebody.com/asp/sept01/peer.html. Accessed on 1/15/05.

A CASE STUDY IN THE USE OF A TAILORED
MAIL-OUT REMINDER

Two separate projects tested the feasibility of using mail-out reminders in the form of birthday cards to influence health behavior. In one project, researchers designed birthday cards and newsletters to encourage smoking cessation. In the other, they developed birthday card reminders that encouraged breast and cervical cancer screening. Both projects targeted low-income African Americans.

In the first study, the cards and newsletters were individually tailored based upon ethnicity, gender, and the individual's readiness to change according to the Stages of Change model. Smokers received either:

- Provider prompting
- Tailored cards and newsletters
- Tailored cards, newsletters and telephone counseling

The tailored cards and newsletters exhibited a highly significant impact on smoking behavior. Thirty-three percent of smokers who received only the tailored cards and letters quit smoking compared to thirteen percent of smokers who received provider prompting and nineteen percent of smokers who received the tailored cards and newsletters and telephone counseling.

In the other study, people who received the tailored birthday cards and newsletters showed higher rates of Pap tests and general cancer screening. A example of the mail-out reminders used is presented below:

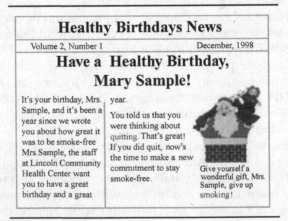

Source: Glassman, B., Rimer, B. K. (1999). "Is there a use for tailored print communications in cancer risk communications?" Monograph of the *Journal of the National Cancer Institute*, No. 25.

A CASE STUDY IN COMMUNICATION STRATEGY

Although more women in recent years have been obtaining mammograms, mammography utilization remains distressingly low. Research has determined that the physician is the most influential factor in a woman's decision to get a mammogram, yet different approaches on the part of physicians are found to yield different results.

Researchers at the University of Kentucky explored strategies available to physicians in promoting mammography. Communication specialists with the AIDS Community Demonstration Project utilized this model to develop and formulate a safer sex campaign for different segments of the female population. Campaign designers determined which internal personal factors were important at the various stages of change, and this information was used to guide message design and intervention tailoring.

While there are numerous message appeals available to practitioners, three are identified here. These message appeals are symbolic messages, instrumental messages, and fear appeal messages. Symbolic messages emphasize the expressive nature of mammograms. Instrumental messages emphasize the direct benefits available to an individual from getting a mammogram. Finally, fear appeal messages raise the threat of breast cancer, but clearly express the effectiveness of mammography as preventive health behavior.

Women in the precontemplation stage are not presently considering mammography utilization, nor do they anticipate acquiring one in the next year. Based on this evidence, it was concluded that lack of knowledge is the primary barrier to mammography utilization for women in the precontemplation stage. This is addressed by making the message detectable and understandable for the woman, while at the same time being considerate of the woman's feelings. One would want the woman's full attention in order to present the information clearly, coherently, and considerately. Here an instrumental or a symbolic message appeal would be an effective means of communicating knowledge. The goal is to offer basic knowledge to the woman about breast cancer and mammography, such that after consideration, hopefully the woman would shift forward one stage of change. Based on the previous evidence, it is believed that these women should be provided with information that goes beyond basic knowledge. The provider should utilize the methods to create awareness and explain difficult ideas.

The model further suggests that women in the preparation stage, on the other hand, are avoiding mammography utilization because of external barriers, primarily related to finances or inconvenience. The most effective means of attaining mammography compliance is by addressing the external barriers of cost, time, and transportation. While women may understand the importance of getting a mammogram and have no fear or shame issues, spending $100 may be quite significant, especially for the uninsured. Given that most facilities prefer payment at the time of service, prioritizing $100 for a mammography instead of for food or clothing for lower income individuals may be a barrier that is difficult to address. Examples related to just two stages underscore the importance of gearing the message to the woman's stage of readiness.

Source: Stephenson, Michael T. (1997). "*Addressing salient barriers in health promotion: A communication framework motivating mammography utilization.*" Presented to the annual meeting of the National Communication Association, Chicago, IL.

A CASE STUDY IN BEHAVIORAL CHANGE

Launched in 1988, the Harvard Alcohol Project sought to demonstrate how a new social concept, the "designated driver," could be rapidly diffused through American society via mass communication, catalyzing a fundamental shift in social norms relating to driving-after-drinking. Such a shift was thought essential for curbing alcohol-related traffic fatalities, the leading cause of death among young adults aged 15–24.

The Harvard Alcohol Project represented a genuine breakthrough for public health. It marked the first time that a health institution joined forces with the communications industry on a project of this magnitude. All major Hollywood studios participated along with the ABC, CBS, and NBC television networks. *Channels*, a respected trade journal, called the extent of this industry involvement "unparalleled," and *The New York Times* lauded the initiative in an editorial.

The Project broke important new ground when TV writers agreed to insert drunk driving prevention messages, including references to designated drivers, into scripts of top-rated television programs, such as "Cheers," "L.A. Law," and "The Cosby Show." The strength of this approach is that short messages, embedded within dialogue, are casually presented by characters who serve as role models within a dramatic context.

At Harvard's request, ABC, CBS, and NBC also aired frequent public service announcements (PSAs) during prime time encouraging the use of designated drivers. This was the first time that the three networks produced and sponsored simultaneous campaigns with the same message. The Center's public relations activities further reinforced the campaign, generating extensive news coverage.

"Designated driver" became a household phrase in the U.S. to such an extent that the term appeared in the 1991 *Random House Webster's College Dictionary*. Public opinion polls documented the rapid, wide acceptance and strong popularity of the designated driver concept. According to the Roper Poll, the proportion of Americans serving as a designated driver reached 37 percent in 1991. Among Americans under the age of 30, 52 percent had actually been a designated driver. Among frequent drinkers, 54 percent had been driven home by a designated driver. Other research found that nearly 9 out of 10 respondents in the country were familiar with the designated driver program.

Source: URL: http://hsph.harvard.edu/chc/alcohol.html Accessed on 1/15/05.

A CASE STUDY IN USING VIDEOS TO REACH YOUTH

A Maryland school district needed a creative approach for reaching youth in order to discourage drug use. They attempted to address this issue through the "Right Turns Only" program. Right Turns Only is a video-based drug education series produced by the Prince George's County, Maryland, school system. The effects of this series (including collateral print material) on student knowledge, attitudes, and behavioral intentions were tested on approximately 1,000 seventh-grade students.

Twelve schools were assigned to one of four groups: three intervention groups and one control group. One intervention group received only the video-based education, a second received both the video-based and a traditional drug education curriculum, a third received only the traditional curriculum, and the control group received no drug abuse prevention education. All interventions were completed within a three-week period.

The six outcomes measured included: 1) knowledge of substance abuse terminology, 2) ability to assess advertisements critically, 3) perception of family, 4) conflict resolution, 5) self-efficacy in peer relationships, and 6) behavioral intentions related to substance use/abuse prevention.

Changes were measured using data from questionnaires completed by students before and after the interventions. The data were analyzed to identify differences based on gender, race, grades (self-reported), and teacher. Groups that received drug education scored higher than the control group on all posttest measures except self-efficacy. On two of the six measures, the group receiving the combination of the video series and traditional curriculum scored significantly higher than other groups.

The evaluation demonstrated that instructional videos (particularly when used in conjunction with print materials and teacher guidance) could be an effective tool for delivering drug education in the classroom.

Source: Center for Substance Abuse Prevention. (1998). Evaluating the results of communication programs (Technical Assistance Bulletin), August. Washington, DC: US Government Printing Office.

A CASE STUDY IN USING EVALUATION TO JUSTIFY A COMMUNICATION PROGRAM

The National Cancer Institute (NCI) evaluated its information dissemination arm, Cancer Information Services (CIS), in order to determine the effectiveness of the program in serving its customers. CIS produced an evaluation report, "Making a Difference," to show its partners, the research community, NCI/CIS leadership, and the media that its programs were effective. The document both quantified CIS results (e.g., making 100,000 referrals a year to research studies, providing information on breast cancer to 76,000 callers in 1996, providing information that increased fruit and vegetable consumption among callers) and put a human face on the calling public. Quotations from callers and leaders in the cancer community illustrated the personal impact of the service on people's lives and health.

CIS surveys of its users indicated among other findings that:

- Eight out of 10 callers said they had taken positive steps to improve their health after talking with CIS staff.
- Seventy percent of those who had called about their symptoms indicated that the CIS information was helpful in their decision to see a doctor.
- Fifty-five percent of those who had called about treatment said they used CIS information to make a treatment decision.
- Two-thirds of callers who were considering participation in a research study talked with a doctor after calling the CIS.

The report was written in lay language and used pullouts and simple charts to explain statistics. Ideas for using the report with regional partners, the media, and community leaders were included with the copies sent to each CIS office. To maximize opportunities for using the report, CIS also made it available on computer disk and as a PowerPoint slide presentation.

A CASE STUDY IN COMMUNICATING WITH HARD-TO-REACH POPULATIONS

One of the challenges in developing prevention programs for syphilis is the difficulty in reaching the at-risk population. Syphilis is not easy to talk about, and it is difficult to engage the community around this particular subject. This is particularly an issue when it comes to hard-to-reach populations. As a result, the Metropolitan Nashville Health Department developed innovative approaches for effectively reaching those at risk of syphilis.

Once the target population had been identified, a number of approaches were utilized, starting with a community blitz. This blitz began with "faith symposiums" to address the issue of denial within the faith community. This was followed by a number of community outreach activities. For World AIDS Day, condoms were handed out and people were tested right there on the spot for HIV and syphilis. Outreach workers were sent to barber and beauty shops carrying little cards with condoms in them and giving customers in these shops invitations to come to the Health Department for free syphilis testing. Outreach workers also went into city parks where at-risk populations tended to congregate. The Syphilis Elimination Kick Off, a national event held in Nashville, was established, using professional athletes as role models for getting tested. Radio "testimonials" were developed to encourage people over the radio to come and get tested at one of the sites.

In order to reach college students, a Haunted House concept was developed to entertain students and to increase their awareness of STDs, help inculcate some skills into the student population, and encourage them to be tested. Skill building involved activities like proper use of a condom. One-on-one counseling was also offered at the Haunted House. "Trick-or-treat" bags with condoms, candy and information were handed out. Evaluations collected from participants in the Haunted House informed the process and the theme has changed every year.

A CASE STUDY IN THE USE OF HEALTH EDUCATION MATERIALS FOR MARKETING

Hospital-sponsored educational sessions are certainly not a new concept, but they can be used as a means to impart information on "hot topics", improve the health of a targeted population, and promote programs and services that are offered by the hospital. Short sessions lasting 1–2 hours offered during the day or in the evening that feature a particular "expert" can be an effective way to advertise a service or build the practice of a new physician. As an example, one hospital provides short sessions on infertility issues to promote the hospital's new fertility program. These sessions are usually free and are advertised in the newspaper, through radio public service announcements (PSA), and on a large billboard hung from the parking structure of the hospital.

Advertisements and promotions raise awareness, but educational events are often the tie that binds an individual to an organization. One hospital developed an annual *Women's Health Symposium*. Initially, the turnout was modest and the event was held on the hospital campus. Because of the quality of the programming, the event grew in reputation and in volume of attendees and was held annually in the community convention center. High-profile speakers started and ended the day and provided lunchtime "info-tainment". Breakout sessions featured a host of age- and stage-specific topics, and an *Ask Your Doctor* corner featured a number of the hospital's more prominent and willing experts in women related health specialties. The participants could obtain advice from the doctor/consultant on any relevant topic. The symposium even included an exhibition hall with community vendors featuring massage therapy, cosmetics, clothing lines, food and nutritional items, exercise related items, and other products of interest to women.

At the end of the symposium, a questionnaire was distributed to obtain feedback related to the overall quality of the symposium, speakers, luncheon food, and the environment. In addition, another strategic question was asked: Does this symposium or other educational sessions offered by this hospital influence your decision to: 1) select Hospital X as your preferred hospital for care; 2) select an insurance carrier that uses Hospital X as a provider; or 3) select a physician that uses Hospital X? Interestingly, over 50 percent of the respondents indicated that they were influenced by the hospital's educational offerings. Of the women who were currently receiving care someplace, nearly one-third of women affiliated with a different hospital system indicated their interest in switching healthcare plans or physicians to come to the hospital that sponsored the annual event and monthly educational offerings.

Women are the decision makers with regard to their family's healthcare. They make decisions as to where they will obtain information and care, and they strongly influence the decisions of family and friends. Carefully planned and presented health education programs on topics of interest to women of all ages and stages of life can be very effective marketing tools and the tie that binds an individual to the hospital or healthcare system that is willing to put forth this effort.

Source: Stichler, Jaynelle, F. (2002). "Strong relationships start with education," *Marketing Health Services*, 22(2), 14–15.

A CASE STUDY IN CONCEPT TESTING

A panel of respondents was used to test the effectiveness of different concepts designed to raise awareness of the need for hearing aids. Three advertising themes were tested in this study: "warm and emotional," "educational," and "wedge of doubt." The *warm and emotional* print advertisement began with text at the top of the page, "Honey, can you pick up some nails?" A response of "Sure" was printed in the middle of the page, with a photograph of a can of escargot. The tag-line printed at the bottom of the page inquired, "Is it any wonder hearing loss can frustrate those around you?... Have your hearing checked. For you. For them."

The text for the *educational* message stated, "Use your head once a year" atop a photograph of headphones. The ad's closing text read: "Annual hearing checkups help you spot changes in your hearing....Hear today. Hear tomorrow."

The *wedge of doubt* advertisement began with text that warned: "If you think it's difficult admitting your hearing problem, imagine admitting all the mistakes you've made because of it." At the bottom, the ad read: "When you can't hear clearly, it's easy to misunderstand someone. And before you know it, people start thinking you've lost your mental edge."

Each of the messages appealed to some segments of the target population. The effectiveness of each of the messages was affected by the type of media that was used to deliver it. These findings demonstrated that rarely can a communicator choose a medium or advertising message without considering the big picture. Thoughtful combinations of media and messages appear to go farther in getting a message across than haphazard collections of media and messages. .

Source: Iacobucci, Dawn, Calder, Bobby J., Malthouse, Edward, and Adam Duhachek (2002). "Did you hear: Consumers tune into multimedia marketing," *Marketing Health Services*, 22(2), 16–20.

A CASE STUDY IN EVALUATING THE COST-EFFECTIVENESS OF COMMUNICATION

When incoming residents relocate to a new community, they have to think about new jobs and schools, new neighbors, new grocery stores and new healthcare providers. To extend a warm welcome to area newcomers and to acquaint them with its healthcare facilities and services, Johnson Memorial Hospital (JMH), in Franklin, Indiana, began a newcomers campaign in January of 2000. The program is part of JMH's ongoing effort to develop lasting relationships with its customers in an area of tremendous population growth. During 2000, the hospital sent packets entitled "Why healthy living is easier in Johnson County" to new residents in its service area. The packet included information about the hospital's call center and physician referral line, a map, service addresses, and a refrigerator magnet to keep the telephone number close at hand.

To reach the right people in the JMH market, the hospital purchased a household list and reduced it to non-duplicated names and addresses. The hospital then matched both the name and address to its admissions and billings records and removed anyone at a "new address" who had previously received service at JMH prior to a specified date.

To encourage responses, the package offered a free first aid kit and a Healthy Living Quiz to recipients who returned a business reply card. During the first year of the program, JMH seat out nearly 5,000 newcomer packets. This initiative ultimately generated 467 hospital encounters—i.e., hospital visits or admissions—from individuals who received the mailing for an unprecedented 10 percent response rate. The gross revenue from these visits and discharges was $368,343, with net revenue totaling $74,000.

The newcomers program start-up and operational program costs were $39,653. The newcomer packets were designed and printed at a total cost of $6,343.75, or $1.27 per piece. Letter shop costs, postage, fulfillment and batch scanning of the Healthy Living Quiz offer brought the total to about $7.93 per new mover. JMH was able to confirm that the hospital's ER and outpatient services are the leading gateway of service to the hospital for new residents, with those areas accounting for 84 percent of the hospital activity generated.

The outstanding results achieved with this program led to an increase in marginal revenue and a decrease in general operating costs, allowing the hospital to put more resources into patient services. The ability to gather new insights into the utilization of hospital services by new residents also was beneficial. Using this database for ROI analysis, JMH was also able to track gross and net revenue by service and identify gross revenue by payer.

Source: Paddison, Nancy V. (2001). "A healthy start," *Marketing Health Services*, 21(3), 31-32.

A CASE STUDY IN COMMUNICATING
WITH REFERRAL AGENTS

With increasing competition in all sectors of the healthcare arena, organizations are constantly seeking new avenues for communicating with important constituents. Clergy represent an untapped target for market collaboration and customer expansion. It is not unusual for members of places of worship to seek advice and counsel from clergy for matters ranging from having a baby, chronic disease management, and dealing with an aging family member to chemical dependency and mental health problems.

Beyond the spiritual visit to a hospitalized or homebound patient, clergy should be considered as part of the healthcare team. Here are some tactics for successfully communicating with clergy:

- Every new clergy person in the community should be invited to an individualized, focused and comprehensive orientation to the healthcare organization. The orientation should cover departments, services and staff that have the most interactions with the clergy, along with facility tours, meetings with executives, and information about programs and activities.

- If the organization has a pastoral care department, a member of that team should be assigned as a "buddy" to the new clergy person. If not, he or she should be assigned to a member of the management team. The "buddy" should guide them through the healthcare maze, making them feel part of the "family" and encouraging them to refer members of their congregation to your organization. This relationship should be ongoing with continuing needs assessments, calls, visits and meetings.
- As major potential referral sources, clergy secretaries and coordinators who interact with members are extremely influential in referrals to health entities. Consider an orientation for these individuals and periodic programs to educate them on new activities and services, as well as how to deal with congregants with health problems and on specific resources available for health-related questions and concerns.
- Include clergy, their staff and key volunteer leaders in your database. With proper information and continued interaction, these "opinion leaders" can influence the healthcare choices of fellow congregants.
- Provide a site for ministerial association meetings and coordinate programming and speakers. Ensure that each session begins with an update of your organization's activities, tips to keep clergy healthy, education on dealing with aging or seriously ill parishoners and more.
- Consider a clergy hot line, a special telephone number that can be answered immediately to respond to clergy questions and concerns.
- Provide links from Web sites of places of worship to your site, especially those areas that deal with health and wellness and list easy-to-access programs and services.
- Offer health-related articles for clergy, places of worship for posting on their Web sites and as information for their newsletters. Provide ongoing communications materials at the place of worship.

As if often the case, marketing opportunities present themselves in unexpected places. When developing a communication plan, clergy and places of worship probably do not come immediately to mind. However, these unlikely targets for healthcare marketing have the potential to pay significant dividends.

Source: Weiss, Rhoda (2002). "New targets offer unexpected rewards," *Marketing Health Services*, 22(3), 10–11.

Chapter 12

Evaluating the Impact of Health Communication

E valuating the effectiveness of a communication initiative is often an afterthought—and this is particularly the case in healthcare. Mechanisms for assessing both the efficiency and effectiveness of a communication campaign must be built into any project on the front-end. This chapter examines the evaluation needs inherent in any communication initiative. The intent of this chapter is not to turn health communicators into evaluators but to expose health professionals to the evaluation process and create an awareness of the importance and nature of this component of the communication initiative.

OVERVIEW OF THE EVALUATION PROCESS

Anyone reflecting on the success of a communication campaign will probably raise a number of obvious questions. One would like to know, for example, how appropriate was the message for the target audience? How effective were the channels utilized? How well did the message reach the target audience? What changes resulted from the communication initiative? To what extent did the campaign achieve its goal(s)? Were the benefits derived from the exercise worth the cost of doing it? These are the types of questions that project evaluation should answer and the type of questions addressed in this chapter.

The evaluation of any communication initiative should be top of mind from the initiation of the project and, in fact, should be built into the methodology itself. Evaluation techniques focus on two types of analysis, although the variety of evaluation options is quite broad. Process (or formative) evaluation assesses the efficiency of the marketing effort, while outcome evaluation addresses its effectiveness. Together, process and outcome evaluation indicate how the program is functioning and why. (It is often the case that organizations do not have adequate evaluation resources in house and have to resort to the use of an outside consultant. See Box 12.1 for a discussion on the use of evaluation consultation.)

Box 12.1

Using Evaluation Expertise

Most organizations involved in health communication do not have the necessary evaluation expertise in house. This may necessitate the use of an evaluation consultant. An evaluation expert familiar with evaluating communication projects should be utilized during initial project planning. His or her advice can help prevent time-consuming fixes later by ensuring a project design that is amenable to evaluation (e.g., making sure data collection mechanisms are in place or making sure baseline data are collected for comparison later).

The more complex the evaluation design, the more expert assistance will be required to conduct the evaluation and interpret the results. The expert can also help write questions that produce objective results.

It order to prepare the evaluation report, appropriate statistical expertise will be required for analyzing the data. One of the major pitfalls in evaluation is generating output that cannot be used for evaluation purposes. All initiatives generate data but these data are not worth much if they do not lend themselves to statistical analysis. Project staff should work closely with the experts in interpreting the data and developing recommendations.

Although there is not a surplus of skilled evaluators, other similar organizations may have used such resources in the past. Other sources of evaluation expertise include university faculty (and their students) and state and local health agencies.

PROCESS EVALUATION

Process evaluation is used to document how well a program has been implemented and to adjust communication activities to meet project objectives. This type of evaluation is used to examine the operations of a program, including which activities are taking place, who is conducting the activities, and who is reached through the activities. Process evaluation assesses whether inputs or resources have been allocated or mobilized and whether activities are being implemented as planned. It involves on-going monitoring of the processes employed, including benchmarks and/or milestones for assessment along the way. It identifies program strengths, weaknesses, and areas that need improvement.

Process evaluation takes place during implementation and monitors the functioning of program components. It includes assessment of whether messages are being delivered appropriately, effectively, and efficiently; whether materials are being distributed to the right people and in the right quantities; and whether the intended program activities are occurring, along with other measures of how well the program is working. (See Box 12.2 for an example of measuring participant satisfaction.)

Box 12.2

Measuring Audience Satisfaction

Audience satisfaction surveys are an important tool for both process and outcome evaluation of health communication programs. Surveys can be used to identify:

- The characteristics of those reached
- How the intended audience reacted to the materials and services
- How the intended audience used the materials

This information will help determine whether the communication is reaching the intended audiences, whether the materials or activities need to be revised, and whether the materials are being used as intended.

Audience satisfaction measurement can be used to assess a completed project or bring about changes in an on-going project. Some managers also use these surveys to learn what information intended audiences would like to receive in the future.

The following are examples of the type of tangible program indicators measured by process evaluation:

- The context in which the communication is carried out
- The number of people exposed to the communication
- The characteristics of people exposed to the communication
- The type and amount of resources expended
- Media response

- Intended audience participation, inquiries, and other responses
- Adherence to schedule
- Meeting of deadlines
- Production of deliverables
- Print coverage and estimated readership
- Quantities of educational materials distributed
- Number of speeches and presentations given
- Number of special events sponsored

OUTCOME EVALUATION

Outcome evaluation is used to assess the effectiveness of a program in meeting its stated objectives. While process evaluation considers how well the process is carried out, outcome evaluation considers the consequences (intended and unintended) of the project. The outcome evaluation plan is developed during the planning phase to identify what changes (e.g., in knowledge, attitudes, or behavior) did or did not occur as a result of the program.This type of evaluation assesses what has occurred because of the program and whether the program has achieved its outcome objectives. Outcome evaluation should be conducted only when the program is mature enough to produce the intended outcome.

Some consider outcome assessment to focus on short- or intermediate-term outcomes, while the assessment of long-term outcomes may be thought of as impact evaluation. *Short-term* outcomes refer to the immediate or early results of the program. These may involve changes in knowledge, attitudes, and skills. *Intermediate* outcomes reflect further progress in reaching a program goal. Intermediate outcomes may involve changes in individual behaviors, social norms, or the environment. *Long-term* outcomes relate to the ultimate goal of the program. The long-term outcome of a program would be something like decreased morbidity as a result of the communication effort.

Decisions as to whether a particular outcome is short-term, intermediate, or long-term depend on the purpose of the program and the time needed for the change to occur.

Outcome evaluations should measure, among other factors, the following:

- Changes in people's attitude and beliefs
- Changes in intended and actual behaviors
- Changes in public and private policies
- Changes in population attributes
- Changes in trends in morbidity and mortality

The following points should be kept in mind as the outcome evaluation is developed:

- Ensure that the evaluation design is appropriate for the particular communication activity.
- Ensure that the activity is evaluated in accordance with expectations with regard to outcomes and timeframes.
- Consider what level of evidence is acceptable for outcome evaluation purpose.
- Consider what baseline measures are available or can be established for tracking changes related to desired outcomes.
- Ensure that change is measured against the communication objectives and not against the program's goal.
- Ensure that *progress* toward outcomes is measured even though objectives may not be completely met.

The following steps should be followed in conducting an outcome evaluation:

1. Determine what information the evaluation must provide.
2. Define the data to be collected.
3. Decide on data collection methods.
4. Develop and pretest data collection instruments.
5. Collect data.
6. Process data.
7. Analyze data to answer the evaluation questions.
8. Write an evaluation report.
9. Disseminate the evaluation report.

The timing of outcome evaluation is an important consideration, since the findings from the evaluation will differ depending on the point at which measure occurs. For example, if it is expected that people will require several exposures to a message before they take action, sufficient implementation time should be allowed to achieve the intended level of exposure. If immediate action is expected after exposure, then the outcome measurement should take place soon after the communication occurs. Conversely, if effects are not expected for at least a year, outcomes should not be measured until then.

IMPACT EVALUATION

Impact evaluation assesses the extent to which a communication campaign induced the desired change (e.g., an increase in consumer approval or greater patient volume). The actual impact of a communication program is often difficult to assess accurately. Can one public service announcement produced by the health department through its social marketing initiative, for example, cause a drop in morbidity and mortality from heart disease? Probably not, but many such efforts combined synergistically may be a contributing factor in health status improvement. Because communication campaigns are relatively short lived, it is impossible to determine the effect of a particular spot on overall trends. However, in this example it would be possible to compare mortality and morbidity rates before and after implementation of the program as one form of measurement.

Information generated through impact evaluation informs decisions on whether to expand, modify, or eliminate a particular policy or program and can be used in prioritizing public actions. In addition, impact evaluation contributes to the effectiveness of policies and programs by addressing the following questions:

- Does the program achieve the intended goal?
- Can the changes in outcomes be explained by the program, or are they the result of some other factors occurring simultaneously?
- Do program impacts vary across different groups of intended audiences, geographic areas, and over time?
- Are there any unintended effects of the program, either positive or negative?
- How effective is the program in comparison with alternative interventions?

The same processes outlined in the previous section should be followed in conducting impact evaluation.

COST ANALYSES

Increasingly, health professionals are being asked to justify a communication initiative in terms of its return on investment (ROI). Not only does this require a carefully constructed communication plan, but it demands detailed record keeping with regard to both the expenditures and revenues associated with a communication initiative. Some type of financial analysis should be conducted prior to the initiation of the project and every effort made to track the benefits that accrue to the organization (in terms of visibility, perception, market share, volume and revenue) as a result of the marketing effort.

The costs associated with a program could be measured through either a cost-benefit analysis or a cost-effectiveness analysis. A cost-benefit analysis is a systematic cataloguing of impacts as benefits (pros) and costs (cons), valuing them in monetary units (assigning weights), and then determining the net benefits of the proposed project or activity relative to the status quo (net benefits equal benefits minus costs).

A cost-effectiveness analysis may be used to assess the comparative impacts of expenditures on different health interventions. It is therefore necessary to define the core concepts of "effectiveness". A very simple definition of effectiveness in health-related activities is that health services are considered to be effective to the extent that they achieve health improvements in real practice settings.

While the outcomes in a cost-effectiveness analysis might not be necessarily expressed in monetary values but in measures such as moral hazard or safe communities, a cost-benefit analysis requires a monetisation of both costs and benefits.

A cost analysis can be targeted toward a single decision-making process or a continuous process, e.g., resource allocations at the societal level. Applied to health-related issues, a cost-effectiveness analysis requires a numerical estimate of the magnitude of the effects of an intervention on health outcomes. It is usually expressed in a cost-effectiveness ratio which is the difference in effectiveness between an intervention and the alternative.

Unlike most other industries, healthcare may embark on initiatives that are not profitable in the normal business sense. They may be designed to generate intangible benefits that may not pay off financial in the short run (or even in long run). This obviously has implications for the approach to evaluation.

EVALUATION TECHNIQUES

The field of health communication is under increasing pressure to demonstrate that programs are worthwhile, effective, and efficient. During the last two decades, our knowledge and understanding about how to evaluate communication projects have increased significantly. The appropriateness of the evaluation design is a primary concern. Different types of evaluation call for different techniques, so it might be helpful to describe some common evaluation designs, the situations in which they are appropriate, and their major limitations. Most evaluation designs are relatively straightforward, although complex, multifaceted programs may employ a range of methods so that each activity is evaluated appropriately. The design selected influences the timing of data collection, the manner in which the data are analyzed, and the types of conclusions that can be drawn from the findings. Most outcome evaluation methods involve collecting data about participants through observation, a questionnaire, or another method. Instruments may include tally sheets for counting public inquiries, survey questionnaires, interview guides. The method chosen should be one that takes into consideration the characteristics of the intended audience and the resources available.

All communication projects should involve process evaluation, and the following are examples of ways to gather the information needed to carry that out:

- Use activity tracking forms
- Monitor the volume of public inquiries and requests for information
- Interview callers who respond to a call-for-action
- Use clipping services to gauge media coverage
- Gather feedback cards from or make follow-up phone calls to television and radio stations
- Gather regular status reports from staff, contractors, and partners
- Meet in person or by telephone with partners to review the program's progress
- Track traffic to project Websites
- Count the requests for information on the subject of the communication initiative
- Have participants maintain diaries or activity logs

The project plan—especially the implementation plan—plays an important part in process evaluation, since it indicates the milestones, benchmarks, and other factors against which to assess the efficiency of the project.

Three general types of outcome evaluation designs are commonly recognized: experimental, quasi-experimental, and observational. Evaluations using experimental designs use random assignment to compare the effect of an intervention on one or more groups with changes in an equivalent group or groups that did not receive the intervention. For example, an evaluation team could select a group of similar schools, then randomly assign some schools to receive a tobacco-use prevention curriculum and other schools to serve as control schools. All schools have the same chance of being selected as an intervention or control school. Because of the "random assignment," the chances are reduced that the control and intervention schools vary in any way that could influence differences in program outcomes. This allows you to attribute change in outcomes to your program.

Experimental designs, in which a treatment group (people exposed to the communication) is compared to a control group (people not exposed to the communication), are the gold standard of outcome evaluation. However, they often cannot be used to assess communication activities, largely because untreated control groups may not exist, particularly for national-, state-, or community-based efforts. Even if people are not exposed to a program's communication, they are likely to be exposed to some communication on the same topic. In these situations, appropriate designs include comparisons between cross-sectional studies (such as independent surveys taken at different points in time), panel studies (the same people are interviewed or observed multiple times), and time series analyses (comparisons between projections of what would have happened without the intervention versus what did happen). This is one of those points at which input from an evaluation expert might be helpful.

Since it is often impossible to utilize an experimental design for evaluating a communication initiative, another option is to use a quasi-experimental design. These designs make comparisons between nonequivalent groups and do not involve random assignment to intervention and control groups. An example would be to assess adults' beliefs about the harmful effects of second-hand smoke in two communities, then conduct a media campaign in one of the communities. After the campaign, you would reassess the adults and expect to find a higher percentage of adults who believe second-hand smoke is harmful in the community that received the media campaign. These types of studies are often used to measure the impact of an intervention that involves communication efforts on members of a health plan or other formally organized groups of individuals to determine the effectiveness of the intervention. Unlike experimental designs, however, it is not possible in this case to control the many variables that might contribute to the observed effects.

Observational designs are also used in program evaluation. These include, but are not limited to, longitudinal, cross-sectional surveys and case studies. Periodic cross-sectional surveys can inform an evaluation. Case studies are often applicable when the program is unique, when an existing program is used in a different setting, when you are assessing a unique outcome, or when an environment is especially unpredictable. Case studies can also allow for an exploration of community characteristics and how these may influence program implementation as well as the identification of barriers to and facilitators of change. (Whatever type of evaluation design is utilized, it should take into consideration the cultural traits of the intended audience. See Box 12.3 for a discussion of culturally competent evaluation.)

REFINING THE HEALTH COMMUNICATION PROGRAM

The implementation stage will not always proceed as expected. Materials may be delayed at the printer, a major news story may preempt your publicity (or focus additional attention on your issue), or a new priority may delay community participation. A periodic review of the planned tasks and time schedules will help you revise any plans that might be affected by unexpected events or delays. It may be necessary to alter the course of the project. The communication initiative should be flexible enough to respond to any identified issues.

As the project progresses it is important to review that plan to ensure it still fits the program. A number of factors will influence how your communication program's outcomes should be evaluated, including the

Box 12.3

Conducting Culturally Competent Evaluation

Any effort at evaluating a communication program involves a set of assumptions about what should happen, to whom, and with what results. These assumptions and expectations will vary depending on the cultural norms and values of the intended audiences. The methods used for evaluation (e.g., for data collection and analysis of the results) may vary depending on the characteristics of the group involved. Depending on the culture from which information is being collected, people may react in the following ways:

- They may think it is inappropriate to speak out in a group, such as a focus group, or to provide negative answers.
- They may be reluctant to provide information to a person from a different culture or over the telephone.
- They may lack familiarity with printed questionnaires or have a limited ability to read English.

For these reasons, careful consideration should be given to the instruments utilized for evaluation of projects with diverse populations.

It should be remembered, as well, that the culture of the evaluator the program uses can inadvertently affect the objectivity of your evaluation. When possible, culturally competent evaluators should be used to examine program activities. If a program cuts across cultures and its becomes necessary to adapt the evaluation methods to fit different groups, it may become difficult to compare results across groups. This is another case where the help of an expert evaluator may be required.

type of communication program, the communication objectives, budget, and timing. The outcome evaluation process needs to capture intermediate outcomes and measure the outcomes specified in the communication objectives.

Since the health communication planning process is circular, the evaluation stage is not the end of the process but should direct project staff back to the beginning. In refining the project plan, the following factors should be considered:

- Goals and objectives
  Have the goals and objectives shifted as the program has progressed?

Are there objectives the program is not meeting?

If so, what are the barriers that are being encountered?

- Additional effort:

Is there new health information that should be incorporated into the program's messages or design?

Are there additional activities that might increase its success?

- Indicators of success

Which objectives have been met, and by what successful activities? Should successful communication activities be continued and strengthened because they appear to work well or should they be considered successful and completed?

Can successful communication activities be expanded to apply to other audiences or situations?

- Costs incurred

What costs have been incurred and how to they relate to different aspects of the program?

Do some activities appear to work as well as but cost less than others?

- Accountability

Is the evidence of program effectiveness adequate to devote resources to continue the program?

Do all appropriate parties appear to be providing the necessary inputs?

Once the above questions have been answered, it is possible to specify new activities, identify expanded or different audiences, and revise the communication plan to accommodate new approaches, new tasks, and new timelines.

Additional Resources

Agency for Toxic Substances and Disease Registry. (1994). *Guidelines for planning and evaluating environmental health education programs.* Atlanta.

Center for Substance Abuse Prevention. (1998). *Evaluating the results of communication programs* [Technical Assistance Bulletin]. Washington, DC: US Government Printing Office.

Muraskin, L. D. (1993). *Understanding evaluation: The way to better prevention programs.* Washington, DC: US Department of Education.

Windsor, R. W., Baranowski, T. B., Clark, N. C., & Cutter, G. C. (1994). *Evaluation of health promotion, health education and disease prevention programs* (2nd ed.). Mountain View, CA: Mayfield.

Chapter 13

The Future of Health Communication

This final chapter reviews anticipated changes in society and healthcare that are expected to have implications for health communication in the future. Anticipated innovations in health communication are described and their implications for the evolution of the field discussed. The future characteristics of health communication and the role of the health communicator in the 21st century are addressed.

DEVELOPMENTS IMPACTING HEALTH COMMUNICATION

A number of changes, many of them discussed in previous chapters, are likely to influence the health communication patterns of the future. The key ones are discussed below.

Developments in Consumer Characteristics

The healthcare consumer continues to evolve and a number of attributes characterize the "new consumer". The future healthcare consumer is likely to be older and wiser than any previous ones. Future consumers will certainly be well educated and better informed on health issues than in the past. Spurred on by the aggressive baby boom cohort and facilitated by modern communications, future healthcare consumers will be increasingly demanding.

The consumer population likely to be targeted by health communicators is becoming increasingly diverse. Rather than becoming more alike,

Americans are becoming more differentiated. Driven by growing immigration and a newfound appreciation of the cultural heritage of various immigrant groups, a large and growing share of the U.S. population needs (and wants) communication tailored to their situation.

One implication of the growing diversity is the possibility of wider disparities within the population when it comes to healthcare. These disparities will present a challenge to health communicators and require creativity in addressing increasingly diverse information needs and communication preferences.

The American consumer is also becoming more technology oriented. This has implications ranging from the type of communication vehicle preferred to the desired source of health information. As noted elsewhere, the population is increasingly wired and the number of Americans without Internet access is dwindling rapidly.

These developments have a number of implications for health communication and will help shape the field. These developments mean that the health communicator must be in closer touch with the end-user than at any time in memory, ultimately developing an in-depth understanding of the wants, needs and preferences of the various categories of potential customers. He must be able to determine who wants particular products and services and the extent to which a population category wants standardization versus customization. This will require the development of an advanced understanding of consumer characteristics and behaviors down to the household level, as is already being done in other industries.

Developments in Healthcare

The development of a national health information infrastructure will have a significant impact on many aspects of health communication. Although an efficient infrastructure is just a "pipe dream" at this point, health professionals need to prepare for the eventuality of much better access to information and more effective ways to accessing the healthcare consumer. Admittedly, there are technical, ethnical and financial issues to be addressed (and in many ways we appear to be losing ground with regard to information management), but the gravity of the situation will eventually result in a much more effective health data management system.

Another development in healthcare is the growing emphasis on measuring return on investment (ROI). Primarily driven by the abuses carried out in the name of healthcare advertising in the past, there is growing concern over the cost-benefit ratio of all healthcare operations including communication. While healthcare will always include a number of intangibles, there is likely to be growing pressure on communicators to make the "business case" for the initiatives they want funded.

The paradigm change that is occurring in healthcare is another consideration when it comes to the future of health communication. The shift from an emphasis on medical care to one on healthcare is setting the healthcare field on its head. This has important implications for the content of health communication and the targets for communication initiatives. As the industry shifts from an emphasis on treatment and cure to one on prevention and health maintenance, the context, messages, audiences and other aspects of health communication can be expected to change. Healthcare marketers are already being asked to address these issues, as they seek out well consumers rather than sick people, discourage consumers from using services rather than encouraging them, and face much different criteria for the determination of the success of their communication efforts.

HEALTH COMMUNICATION REQUIREMENTS

For health communication to contribute to the improvement of personal and community health during the first decade of the 21st century, stakeholders, including health professionals, researchers, public officials, and the lay public, must collaborate on a range of activities. These activities include:

- Initiatives to build a robust health information system that provides equitable access
- The development of high-quality, audience-appropriate information and support services for specific health problems and health-related decisions for all segments of the population, especially underserved persons
- The training of health professionals in the science of communication and the use of communication technologies
- Improved evaluation of interventions
- The promotion of a critical understanding and the practice of effective health communication

In addition to these requirements, health communicators will be required to take a more interdisciplinary approach to information transfer. The healthcare field is already overwhelmingly complex and is only going to become more so. Add to this the increasingly diverse audiences for health communication and the situation becomes particularly challenging. The health communication field must draw more heavily from the social sciences, especially in terms of their insights into health behavior and attitudes. The health communicator must be knowledgeable about a wide range of clinical issues, an already complicated situation made worse by emerging ethical issues in healthcare. (The Healthy People 2010 program

developed by federal healthcare officials lays out objectives for the next
several years in the area of health communication in Box 13.1.)

Box 13.1

Healthy People 2010 Objectives

The future of health communication will inevitably be guided to
some extent by federal policies. The primary federal initiative related to
health policy is built around the Healthy People 2010 program. Among
the hundreds of Healthy People objectives, six deal specifically with
health communication. The following general objectives have been set
out for the year 2010:

11-1. Increase the proportion of households with access to the Internet
at home.
11-2. Improve the health literacy of persons with inadequate or
marginal literacy skills.
11-3. Increase the proportion of health communication activities that
include research and evaluation.
11-4. Increase the proportion of health-related World Wide Web sites
that disclose information that can be used to assess the quality
of the site.
11-5. Increase the number of centers of excellence that seek to advance
the research and practice of health communication.
11-6. Increase the proportion of persons who report that their healthcare providers have satisfactory communication skills.

HEALTH COMMUNICATION CHALLENGES

As a result of the changes that are occurring in society and in healthcare, health communicators face a number of challenges. As can be seen
from the earlier discussion, health communicators face a tremendous challenge in keeping up with changing consumer characteristics. The changing
character of the American consumer independent of the influence of major
waves of immigration makes for a constantly restructured configuration
of consumer characteristics. Changing preferences in communication contexts, sources, messages, and timing all contribute to this challenge. Even
the terminology used to communicate is an issue. Consider the effort that
HIV/AIDS educators have to expend just to keep up with the street terminology utilized by their intended audiences. The use of "last year's" slang
term probably spells doom for a health communication initiative.

   The health communicator also faces the challenge of balancing massi-
fication and customization approaches. There is pressure to get healthcare
messages out to the broadest possible audience, despite the often inefficient
nature of such an approach. There is the conflicting pressure to customize
materials for specific individuals. Fortunately, with today's technology it
is possible to obtain the benefits of mass marketing while also focusing
on targeted subgroups. This means that health communicators must really
know their audiences and be well schooled in the approaches available to
reach the masses in a tailored manner.

   Health communicators will also be faced with the challenge, as noted
above, of "bottom line" accounting. In the past, communication initiatives
were launched because everyone agreed that it was the right thing to do.
There may or may not have been information indicating that this was the
most effective approach. In the future, consensus opinion will not be nearly
as important as being able to demonstrate that a communication initiative
is both effective and cost effective.

   Perhaps the greatest challenge facing health communicators—
especially in light of the above passages—is the need for sound research
and evaluation approaches. Meaningful research and evaluation should
not be afterthoughts but integral parts of initial program design. Research
provides the ideas and tools to design and carry out formative, and outcome evaluation to improve health communication efforts, certify the degree of change that has occurred, and identify programs or elements of
programs that are not working. These processes generate information that
can be used to refine the design, development, implementation, adoption,
redesign, and overall quality of a communication intervention.

   Most programs funded by federal, philanthropic, and not-for-profit
organizations have established requirements for a minimum set of evaluation activities and specific measurements. The level of research and evaluation required should reflect the costs, scope, and potential impact (in
terms of benefit or harm) of the communication activity proposed. At a
minimum, programs should be expected to conduct appropriate audience
testing for need, cultural and linguistic competence, comprehension, and
receptivity. Requirements and specifications for evaluation must be set
for grant-funded communication programs and included in requests for
funding proposals and grant program guidelines as well as for programs
directly funded and implemented by public or private sector organizations
by including research and evaluation activities in their work plans.

   To enlarge the knowledge base of health communication and incorporate it into health promotion practice, a research and training infrastructure
is needed to develop, model, and coordinate activities. One vision calls for
centers of excellence located in academic institutions, national organizations, or research centers to meet scientific and practical needs. The centers would be responsible for an array of activities, such as (1) promoting

the adoption of health communication theories and practices in health-care, disease prevention, and health promotion initiatives, (2) developing and disseminating quality standards, (3) coordinating initiatives to develop a consensus research agenda, (4) developing systems to identify and assess health communication research, (5) evaluating communication strategies, messages, materials, and resources, (6) fostering networking and collaboration among health communicators, health educators, and other health professionals, (7) promoting health communication skills training for health professionals, and (8) promoting research and dissemination activities among specific population groups.

These centers should also provide expert staff, model curricula with core competencies in health communication and media technologies, appropriately equipped media labs, research seminars, continuing education and distance learning courses, and training and placement programs to expand the pool of health communication professionals and health professionals with communication skills. The centers also could create databases that would catalog examples of evaluation studies and reports and collaborate in the dissemination of evaluation information.

INTERFACING HEALTH COMMUNICATION WITH OTHER EFFORTS

Health communication is a critical component of efforts to improve personal and public health. For individuals, effective health communication can help raise awareness of health risks and solutions, provide the motivation and skills needed to reduce these risks, help them find support from other people in similar situations, and affect or reinforce attitudes. Health communication also can increase the demand for appropriate health services and play an important role in helping consumers make complex choices, such as selecting health plans, care providers, and treatments. For the community, health communication can be used to influence the public agenda, advocate for policies and programs, promote positive changes in the socioeconomic and physical environments, improve the delivery of health services, and encourage lifestyles that benefit health and quality of life.

Health communication alone, however, cannot change systemic problems related to health, such as lack of access to healthcare; poverty, discrimination, and prejudice; and lack of needed services. Comprehensive health communication programs should include a systematic exploration of all the factors that contribute to health and the strategies that could be used to influence these factors. Well-designed health communication activities help individuals better understand their needs and their communities' needs, so appropriate actions can be taken to maximize health. Public education campaigns seek to change the social climate to encourage healthy behaviors, create awareness, change attitudes, and motivate individuals to adopt recommended behaviors.

SUMMARY

As patients and consumers become more knowledgeable about health information, services, and technologies, health professionals will need to meet the challenge of becoming better communicators and more effective users of information technologies. Health professionals need a high level of interpersonal skills to interact with diverse populations and patients who may have different cultural, linguistic, educational, and socioeconomic backgrounds. Health professionals also need more direct training in and experience with all forms of computer and telecommunication technologies. In addition to searching for information, patients and consumers want to use technology to discuss health concerns, and health professionals need to be ready to respond. To support an increase in health communication activities, research and evaluation of all forms of health communication will be necessary to build the scientific base of the field and the practice of evidence-based health communication. Collectively, these opportunities represent important areas for making significant improvements in personal and community health.

Additional Resources

US Department of Health and Human Services. (2001). *Healthy People 2010: Lesbian, gay, bisexual, and transgender health.* Washington, DC: US Government Printing Office.
US Department of Health and Human Services. (2000). *Healthy People 2010.* Washington, DC: US Government Printing Office.

Bibliography

Academy for Educational Development. (1995). *A tool box for building health communication capacity*. Washington, DC.

Ad Hoc Committee on Health Literacy for the Council on Scientific Affairs, American Medical Association. (1999). Health literacy: Report of the council on scientific affairs. *JAMA*, 281, 552–557.

Agency for Toxic Substances and Disease Registry. (1994). *Guidelines for planning and evaluating environmental health education programs*. Atlanta: Centers for Disease Control and Prevention.

Andreasen, A. (1995). *Marketing social change: Changing behavior to promote health, social development, and the environment*. San Francisco: Jossey-Bass.

Atkin, C., and Wallack, L., (eds.). (1990). *Mass communication and public health*. Newbury Park, CA: Sage Publications.

Backer, T. E., Rogers, E. M., & Sopory, P. (1992). *Designing health communication campaigns: What works?* Newbury Park, CA: Sage Publications.

Baker, D. W., Parker, R. M., Williams, M. V., et al. (1996). The health care experience of patients with low literacy. *Arch Fam Med*, 5, 329–334.

Baker, D. W., Parker, R. M., Williams, M. V., Clark, W. S. (1998). Health literacy and the risk of hospital admission. *J Gen Intern Med*, 13, 791–798.

Baker, D. W., Parker, R. M., Williams, M. V., et al. (1997). The relationship of patient reading ability to self-reported health and use of health services. *American Journal of Public Health*, 87, 1027–1030.

Berkowitz, Eric N. (1996). *Essentials of health care marketing*. Gaithersburg, MD: Aspen Publishers.

Berkowitz, Eric N., and Hillestad, Steven G. (1991). *Healthcare marketing plans: From strategy to action*. Boston: Jones and Bartlett.

Calvert, P., ed. (1996). *The communicator's handbook: Tools, techniques, and technology* (3rd ed.). Gainesville, FL: Maupin House.

Census Bureau, US Department of Commerce, Washington, DC. "American Factfinder" at URL: http://census.gov. Accessed on 4/15/03.

Centers for Disease Control and Prevention. (1996). *The prevention marketing initiative: Applying prevention marketing* (CDC Publication No. D905). Atlanta: Centers for Disease Control and Prevention.

Center for Substance Abuse Prevention. (1998). *Evaluating the results of communication programs* [Technical Assistance Bulletin]. Washington, DC: US Government Printing Office.

Centers for Disease Control and Prevention. (2000). *Beyond the brochure* (CDC Publication No. PDF-821K). Atlanta: Centers for Disease Control and Prevention.

Davis, T. C., Meldrum, H., Tippy, P. K. P., et al. (1996). How poor literacy leads to poor healthcare. *Patient Care*, 94–108.

Doak, C. C., Doak, L. G., & Root, J. H. (1996). *Teaching patients with low literacy skills.* (2nd ed.). Philadelphia, PA: J.B. Lippincott Company.

Eisenberg, D., & R. C. Kessler. (1993). Unconventional medicine in the United States. *New England Journal of Medicine*, 328, 246–252.

Eng, T. R., Maxfield, A., Patrick, K., et al. (1998). Access to health information and support: A public highway or a private road? *Journal of the American Medical Association*, 280(15), 1371–1375.

Gazmararian, J. A., Baker, D. W., Williams, M. V., et al. (1999). Health literacy among Medicare enrollees in a managed care organization. *Journal of the American Medical Association*, 281, 545–551.

Glanz, K., Lewis, F. M., & Rimer, B. K., (eds.). (1997). *Health behavior and health education: Theory, research, and practice* (2nd ed.). San Francisco: Jossey-Bass.

Glanz, K., & Rimer, B. K. (1995). *Theory at a glance: A guide for health promotion practice* (NIH Publication No. 97–3896). Bethesda, MD: National Cancer Institute.

Green, L. W., & Kreuter, M. W. (1999). *Health promotion planning: An educational and ecological approach.* (3rd ed.). Mountain View, CA: Mayfield Publishing Company.

Harris, L. M., ed. (1995). Health and the new media. *Technologies transforming personal and public health.* Mahwah, NJ: Lawrence Erlbaum Associates.

The Institute of Medicine. (2004). *Crossing the quality chasm: A new health system for the 21st century.* Washington: National Academies Press.

Jackson, L. D., and Duffy, B. K., (eds.). (1998). *Health communication research.* Westport, CT: Greenwood.

Janz, N. K., & Becker, M. H. (1984). The health belief model: A decade later. *Health Education Quarterly*, 11, 1–47.

Kotler, P., & Roberto, E. L. (1989). *Social marketing: Strategies for changing public behavior.* New York: Free Press.

Kreuter, M. W., Strecher, V. J., & Glassman, B. (1999). One size does not fit all: The case for tailoring print materials. *Society of Behavioral Medicine*, 21, 276–283.

Lalonde, B., Rabinowitz, P., Shefsky, M. L., et al. (1997). La Esperanza del Valle: Alcohol prevention novelas for Hispanic youth and their families. *Health Education & Behavior*, 24, 587–602.

Lefebvre, R. C. (2000). Theories and models in social marketing. In P. N. Bloom & G. T. Gundlach, eds., *Handbook of Marketing and Society.* Thousand Oaks, CA: Sage.

Lefebvre, R. C., and Rochlin, L. Social marketing. In: K. Glanz, F. M. Lewis, and B. K. Rimer, eds. (1997). *Health behavior and health education: Theory, research, and practice,* (2nd ed.). San Francisco, CA: Jossey-Bass Publishers, 384–401.

Maibach, E., and Parrott, R. L. (1995). *Designing health messages.* Thousand Oaks, CA: Sage Publications.

Maslow, Abraham. (1970). *Motivation and personality* (2nd ed.). New York: Harper & Row.

Muraskin, L. D. (1993). *Understanding evaluation: The way to better prevention programs.* Washington, DC: U.S. Department of Education.

National Cancer Institute. (2003). *Making health communications work.* Washington, DC: US Department of Health and Human Services (HHS).

National Cancer Institute. (1995). *Clear & simple: Developing effective print materials for low-literate readers* (Pub. No. NIH 95–3594). Washington, DC: HHS.

National Center for Health Statistics. (2002). *Health United States, 2002*. Washington, DC: US Government Printing Office.

Northouse, L. L., and Northouse, P. G. (1998). *Health communication: Strategies for health professionals* (3rd ed.). Stamford, CT: Appleton & Lange.

Omran, A. R. (1971). The epidemiologic transition: A theory of the epidemiology of population change. *Milbank Memorial Quarterly*, 49, 515ff.

Ong, L. M. L., de Haes, J. C. J. M., Hoos, A. M., et al. (1995). Doctor-patient communication: A review of the literature. *Social Science and Medicine*, 40, 903–918.

Piotrow, P. T., Kincaid, D. L., Rimon, II, J. G., et al. (1997). *Health communication*. Westport, CT: Praeger.

Rice, R. E., & Atkin, C. K. (2000). *Public communication campaigns* (3rd ed.). Thousand Oaks, CA: Sage.

Robinson, T. N., Patrick, K., Eng, T. R., et al., (1998). An evidence-based approach to interactive health communication: A challenge to medicine in the Information Age. *Journal of the American Medical Association*, 280, 1264–1269.

Rogers, E. M. (1983). *Diffusion of innovations* (3rd ed.). New York: Free Press.

Rosenberg, E. E., Lussier, M. T., & Beaudoin, C. (1997). Lessons for clinicians from physician-patient communication literature. *Archives of Family Medicine*, 6, 279–283.

Roter, D. L., and Hall, J. A. (1992). *Doctors talking with patients/patients talking with doctors: Improving communication in medical visits*. Westport, CT: Auburn House.

Science Panel on Interactive Communication and Health. T. R. Eng, and D. H. Gustafson, eds. (1999) *Wired for health and well-being: The emergence of interactive health communication*. Washington, DC: HHS.

Scott, S. A., Jorgensen, C. M., & Suarez, L. (1998). Concerns and dilemmas of Hispanic AIDS information seekers: Spanish-speaking callers to the CDC National AIDS hotline. *Health Education & Behavior*, 25(4), 501–516.

Simons-Morton, B. G., Donohew, L., & Crump, A. D. (1997). Health communication in the prevention of alcohol, tobacco, and drug use. *Health Education & Behavior*, 24, 544–554.

Street, R. L., Gold, W. R., & Manning, T., eds. (1997). *Health promotion and interactive technology: Theoretical applications and future directions*. Mahwah, NJ: Lawrence Erlbaum Associates.

Thomas, Richard K. (2004). *Marketing health services*. Chicago: Health Administration Press.

Thornton, Barbara C., and Gary L. Kreps. (1992). *Perspectives on health communication*. Long Grove, IL: Waveland Press.

Ting-Toomey, Stella, (ed.). (1994). *Challenge of facework: Cross-cultural and interpersonal issues*. Albany, NY: State University of New York Press.

US Department of Commerce. (1999). *Falling through the net: Defining the digital divide*. Washington, DC: National Telecommunications and Information Administration, 1999. URL: <http:// ntia.doc.gov/ntiahome/digitaldivide/>July 29.

US Department of Health and Human Services, National Institutes of Health, National Library of Medicine (NLM). (2000). In C. R. Seiden, M. Zorn, S. Ratzan, et al., eds. *Health literacy, January 1990 through 1999*. NLM Pub. No. CBM 2000–1. Bethesda, MD: NLM, February, vi.

US Department of Health and Human Services. (2000). *Healthy People 2010*. Washington: US Government Printing Office.

US Department of Health and Human Services. (2001). *Healthy People 2010: Lesbian, gay, bisexual, and transgender Health*. Washington, DC: US Government Printing Office.

US Office of Disease Prevention and Health Promotion. (2004). Health communication. *Healthy People 2010* (vol. 1). URL: http://healthypeople.gov/Document/HTML/volume1/11HealthCom.htm#_edn4. Accessed on 9/20/04.

Weinreich, Nedra Kline. (1999). *Hands-on social marketing: A step-by-step guide*. Thousand Oaks, CA: Sage.

Weiss, B. D., Blanchard, J. S., McGee, D. L., et al. (1994). Illiteracy among Medicaid recipients and its relationship to health care costs. *Journal of Health Care for the Poor and Under-served*, 5, 99–111.

Williams, M. V., Baker, D. W., Parker, R. M., et al. (1998). Relationship of functional health literacy to patients' knowledge of their chronic disease. A study of patients with hypertension and diabetes. *Archives of Internal Medicine*, 158, 166–172.

Williams, M. V., Baker, D. W., Honig, E. G., et al. (1998). Inadequate literacy is a barrier to asthma knowledge and self-care. *Chest*, 114, 1008–1015.

Windsor, R. W., Baranowski, T. B., Clark, N. C., & Cutter, G. C. (1994). *Evaluation of health promotion, health education and disease prevention programs* (2nd ed.). Mountain View, CA: Mayfield.

Wright, A. L., Naylor, A., Wester, R., et al. (1997). Using cultural knowledge in health promotion: Breastfeeding among the Navajo. *Health Education & Behavior*, 24, 625–639.

Glossary

Accuracy: Content that is valid and without errors of fact, interpretation, or judgment.

Advertising: Any paid form of non-personal presentation and promotion of ideas, goods or services by an identifiable sponsor transmitted via mass media for purposes of achieving marketing objectives.

Agency: An internal or external entity that supports some or all aspects of an organization's communication effort.

Advocacy: Communication directed at policymakers and decision makers to promote policies, regulations, and programs to bring about change.

Attention: A pretesting measure used to describe a message's ability to attract listener or viewer attention; this is often measured as "recall" of a message or image.

Attitude: An individual's predisposition toward an issue, person, or group, which influences his or her response to be positive or negative, favorable or unfavorable.

Availability: Content (whether a targeted message or other information) that is delivered or placed where the audience can access it.

Audience: The set of people, households, or organizations that read, view, hear or are otherwise exposed to a promotional message; the target for a marketer's message.

Balance: Content that fairly and accurately presents the benefits and risks of potential actions or recognizes different and valid perspectives on an issue.

Banner ad: An advertisement involving small "banners" that appear in a newspaper or on a Web page.

Baseline study: The collection and analysis of data regarding an intended audience or situation prior to intervention.

Bounceback card: A short questionnaire, often on a business-reply postcard, that is distributed with materials to collect process evaluation data.

Brand: A concept involving a name, symbol or other identifier used to identify a seller's goods and/or services and differentiate them from similar goods and/or services offered by competitors.

Branding: The process of creating a "brand" for a company, service or product. A brand consists of a name, term, design, symbol, or any other feature that identifies one seller's product(s) as distinct from those of other sellers.

Call center: A centralized communication center established by a healthcare organization for purposes of capturing incoming customer inquiries and generating out-going marketing messages.

Call to action: A statement, usually at the end of a marketing piece, encouraging members of the audience to take action with regard to the good or service being promoted.

Center for Disease Control and Prevention (CDC): The federal agency charged with monitoring morbidity and mortality in the U.S.

Census Bureau: The agency within the U.S. Department of Commerce responsible for the conduct of the decennial census and other data collection activities.

Central-location intercept interviews: A method used for pretesting messages and materials involving "intercepting" potential intended audience members at a highly trafficked location.

Channel: The route of message delivery (e.g., mass media channels; interpersonal channels that include health professional to patient; and community channels).

Client: A type of customer that consumes services rather than goods; in advertising, the entity either internal or external to the marketing organization that is the customer for the promotional project.

Closed-ended questions: Questions that provide respondents with a list of possible answers from which to choose; also called multiple choice, forced-choice, or fixed-choice questions.

Comprehension: A pretesting measure used to determine whether messages are clearly understood.

Comarketing: An approach to marketing in which two or more organizations combine their efforts in the joint pursuit of their individual objectives.

Community outreach: A form of marketing that seeks to present the programs of the organization to the community and establish relationships with community organizations.

Consumer: From a healthcare perspective, any individual or organization within the population that is a potential purchaser of healthcare goods or services.

Consumer behavior: The patterns of consumption of goods and services that characterize healthcare consumers, along with the factors that contribute to this behavior and processes that lead up to a purchase decision.

Consumerism: A movement in healthcare in which healthcare consumers take a more aggressive role in defining their healthcare needs and the manner in which these needs should be met.

Consistency: Refers to content that remains internally consistent over time and also is consistent with information from other sources.

Consumer health information: Information designed to help individuals understand their health and make health-related decisions for themselves and their families.

Consumer panel: A research study in which the buying behavior or other characteristics of a group of consumers are studied over time.

Convenience samples: Respondents selected for interviewing that consist of individuals who are typical of the intended audience and who are easily accessible (e.g., participants at a health fair).

Cost-benefit analysis: Process through which the benefits of an initiative are assessed relative to the costs involved in carrying out the initiative.

Cost-effectiveness analysis: Process through which the effectiveness of an initiative is assessed relative to the costs involved in carrying out the initiative.

Creative brief: A short (one- to two-page) version of the communication strategy statement used to guide development of materials and activities.

Creative department: The component of the marketing department responsible for copy, graphics and creative content.

Cross-selling: A marketing approach through which existing customers are encouraged to buy additional products and services.

Cultural competence: The design, implementation, and evaluation process that accounts for special issues of select population groups (ethnic and racial, linguistic) as well as differing educational levels and physical abilities.

Culture: The way of life of a society that reflects its particular worldview; the tangible and intangible aspects of society that reflect its beliefs, values and norms.

Customer: The purchaser of a good or service; the end-user of a good or service.

Customer relationship management: A business strategy designed to optimize profitability, revenue and customer satisfaction by focusing on customer relationships rather than transactions.

Customer satisfaction: A concept measured in various ways that refers to the level of satisfaction with a good or service produced in a customer.

Database marketing: The establishment and exploitation of data on past and current customers together with future prospects, structured to allow for implementation of effective marketing strategies.

Demand: The extent to which a target population needs and/or wants a particular product.

Demographics: The range of biosocial and sociocultural attributes of a population that influence the communication process.

Decision-making: The process through which consumers determine they have a need for a product, evaluate the available options, and make a choice with regard to a particular product.

Descriptive research: A form of research that involves the development of a profile of the community or population being examined, thereby describing but not explaining the phenomenon.

Direct marketing: A form of marketing that targets specific groups or individuals with specific characteristics and subsequently transmits promotional messages directly to them.

Direct-to-consumer: marketing: An approach to marketing that targets the individual end-user rather than referral agents or intermediaries.

Display advertising: A promotional approach that makes use of posters, billboards, and other signs to present a product to the public.

Early adopter: An individual or group in society that is willing to try new products and services before they are accepted by the general public.

Education Entertainment: A form of health communication in which educational content and information is intentionally incorporated into an entertainment format (e.g., songs, comics, non-news television or radio programming, movies).

Effective market: The portion of the potential business within a specified market area that is considered capturable.

Electronic media: Any form of media in which the message is conveyed electronically, to primarily include radio, television, and the Internet.

End user: The person or organization that ultimately consumes a good or service, regardless of who makes the purchase decision or pays for the product.

Enrollee: An individual who is enrolled in a health plan.

Environmental assessment: A systematic process of data collection and analysis for purposes of profiling and evaluating the external environment faced by an organization.

Environmental factors: Factors that are external to an individual but can influence the individual's behavior (e.g., policies, access to services, geography, physical features).

Ethical evaluation: An approach to evaluation that emphasizes the marketer's responsibility and accountability to the target audience.

Evaluation: The systematic assessment of the efficiency and effectiveness of a particular initiative.

Exploratory research: A form of research aimed at discerning the general nature of the problem or opportunity under study and identifying the associated factors of importance.

Focus group: A qualitative research technique in which an experienced moderator guides about 8 to 10 participants through a discussion of a selected topic used to identify previously unknown issues or concerns or to explore reactions to potential actions, benefits, or concepts during the planning and development stages.

Formative evaluation: Evaluation activities that measure the efficiency of the project; process evaluation.

Formative research: A form of evaluation that assesses the nature of the problem, the needs of the target audience, and the implementation process in order to inform and improve program design.

Frequency: The average number of times an audience is exposed to a specific media message.

Gatekeeper: An organization or individual through which an intended audience can be reached (e.g., an organization, a schoolteacher, a television public service director).

Goal: The generalized outcome a communication initiative hopes to effect.

Government relations: A process through which healthcare organizations maintain liaison with the government agencies that regulate them, determine reimbursement levels, provide funding and otherwise affect their status.

Health belief model: A conceptual framework of health behavior stating that health behavior is a function of both knowledge and motivation.

Health communication: The art and technique of informing, influencing, and motivating individual, institutional, and public audiences about important health issues.

Health education: Any planned combination of learning experiences designed to predispose, enable, and reinforce voluntary behavior conducive to health in individuals, groups, or communities.

Health literacy: The degree to which an individual has the capacity to obtain, process, and understand basic the health information and services needed to make appropriate health decisions.

Health promotion: Any planned combination of educational, political, regulatory, and organizational supports for actions and conditions of living conducive to the health of individuals, groups, or communities.

Hierarchy of needs: The hierarchical prioritization of personal needs ranging from basic survival needs at the bottom of the hierarchy to self-actualization needs at the top.

HIPAA:

The Health Insurance Portability and Account-ability Act that limits access to "protected health information" on individuals.

Image:

The perception of a company, product or service that emphasizes subjective attributes rather than objective attributes (e.g., a caring hospital rather than a well-staffed hospital).

Impact evaluation:

A type of research designed to identify whether and to what extent a program contributed to accomplishing its stated goals.

Implementation plan:

A plan accompanying the communication plan that lays out the process for accomplishing the objectives specified in the plan.

In-depth interviews:

A type of qualitative research in which a trained interviewer guides an individual through a discussion of a selected topic, allowing the person to talk freely and spontaneously.

Intended audience:

The audience selected for program messages and materials. The primary intended audience consists of those individuals the program is designed to affect. The secondary intended audience is the group (or groups) that can help reach or influence the primary audience.

Intended population:

A broad definition of the audience for a program. The intended population is defined by the epidemiology of the problem and factors contributing to it (e.g., women ages 40 and over for a mammography screening program).

Interactive health communication:

The interaction of an individual with an electronic device or communication technology to access or transmit health information or to receive guidance on a health-related issue.

Integrated marketing:

An approach to marketing that involves a level of consistency within the promotional strategy and achieves synergy between its component parts.

Internal marketing: Efforts by a service provider to effectively train and motivate its customer-contact employees and all the supporting service personnel to work as a team to generate customer satisfaction.

Internet: A global network connecting millions of computers all over the world, allowing for the expeditious exchange of information.

Internet marketing: A marketing approach that utilizes the Internet as a means of promoting an idea, organization, service or good.

Literacy: The ability to read, write, and speak in English and to compute and solve problems at levels of proficiency necessary to function on the job and in society, to achieve one's goals, and develop one's knowledge and potential.

Low-intensity marketing: Promotional activities that involve low-cost, relatively unobtrusive marketing techniques (e.g., banner ads).

Low literacy: A limited ability to use printed and written information to function in society, to achieve one's goals, and to develop one's knowledge and potential.

Mail interview: A data collection technique that involves the distribution of a survey instrument via the mail to a predetermined set of respondents who subsequently return the completed questionnaires via the mail.

Market: A real or virtual setting in which potential buyers and potential sellers of a good or service come together for the purpose of exchange.

Market share: The percentage of the total market for a product/service category that has been captured by a particular product/service or by a company that offers multiple products/services in that category.

Marketing: The process of planning and executing the conception, pricing, promotion, and distribution of ideas, goods, and services to create exchanges that satisfy individual and organizational objectives (American Marketing Association).

Marketing brief: A brief document developed for use by a marketing agency or consultant that presents the specifics of the campaign to the extent that they are known.

Marketing budget: The itemization of the resources allocated for a global marketing effort or a specific marketing campaign.

Marketing mix: The proportionate roles that product, price, place and promotion play in the marketing of a particular good or service.

Marketing research: The function that links the consumer, customer, and public to the marketer through information used to identify and define marketing opportunities and problems, generate, refine, and evaluate marketing actions, monitor marketing performance, and improve the understanding of the marketing process.

Mass marketing: A marketing approach that targets the total population as if it were one undifferentiated mass of consumers, usually using broad-based approaches such as network television or newspapers.

Media advocacy: The strategic use of mass media to reframe issues, shape public discussion, or build support for a policy, point of view, or environmental change.

Media buying: The marketing function that involves the researching, selecting and negotiation of media exposure to support a communication effort.

Media literacy: Having the skills to deconstruct media messages to identify the sponsor's motives and to construct or compose media messages representing the intended audience's point of view.

Media plan: A plan developed for a communication initiative that outlines the objectives of the promotional campaign, the target audience, and the specific media vehicles that will be used to reach that audience.

Media supplier: Any of the commercial television companies, commercial radio companies, newspapers and magazine owners, poster companies, and other organizations that make media available to a campaign.

Message: The formal presentation of the information that the communicator is trying to convey; the content of a promotional piece.

Message concepts: Brief statements, sometimes accompanied by visuals, that present key aspects of the communication strategy (e.g., action to be taken, benefit promised in exchange, support for the benefit) to the intended audience.

Micro-marketing: An approach to marketing that breaks the market down to the household or even the individual level in an attempt to target those most likely to consume a product.

Mission: The overarching goal of an organization; its reason for being.

Need: A condition of an individual that indicates the need for a health service; an objective determination of medical necessity.

Networking: The process of establishing and nurturing relationships with individuals and organizations with which mutually beneficial transactions might be carried out.

Niche: A segment of a market that can be carved out based on the uniqueness of the target population, the geographical area or the product.

Not-for-profit: An organization that has been granted tax exempt status by the Internal Revenue Service for purposes of performing certain functions.

Objective: A formally designated achievement to be accomplished in support of a goal that is specific, concise and time-bound.

Outcome: Generally refers to the consequences of a clinical episode (e.g., cure, death).

Outcome evaluation: A form of evaluation that examines the results of a communication intervention, including changes in awareness, attitudes, beliefs, actions, professional practices, policies, costs, and institutional or social systems.

Over-recruiting: Recruiting more survey respondents than required to compensate for expected "no-shows."

Packaging: The presentation of a good or service in terms of physical attributes or the positioning of the product.

Patient: An individual who has been officially diagnosed with a health condition and has subsequently presented himself for formal medical care.

Payer (or payor) mix: The combination of payment sources characterizing a population of patients or consumers; the relative proportions of private insurance, government insurance, and self-pay characterizing a population.

Personal interview: A data collection technique that involves the administration of a survey instrument through face-to-face interaction between the interviewer and the respondent.

Personal sales:	The oral presentation of promotional material in a conversation with one or more prospective purchasers for the purpose of making sales.
Place:	The point of distribution of a healthcare good or service.
Positioning:	The placement of an idea, organization or product in the minds of the market relative to its competition.
Pretesting:	A type of formative evaluation that involves systematically gathering intended audience reactions to messages and materials before the messages and materials are produced in final form.
Price:	The amount of money that is charged for a product (e.g., doctor's fee, insurance premium).
Primary research:	The direct collection of data for a specific use.
Print media:	Any mechanism for delivering a message that utilizes the printed word, such as newspapers, magazines, journals, and newsletters.
Probe:	A technique used primarily in qualitative research (e.g., focus groups, in-depth interviews) to solicit additional information about a question or issue.
Process evaluation:	Research conducted to document and study the functioning of different components of program implementation; includes assessments of whether materials are being distributed to the right people and in what quantities, whether and to what extent program activities are occurring, and other measures of how and how well the program is working.
Product:	Generally thought of as a "good" or a "service" but also including ideas or organizations, the product is the object of the marketer's promotional activities.

Product advertising: Advertising efforts designed to promote specific goods and services rather than the organization overall.

Program objectives: The specific outcomes that you expect your entire program to achieve. These will be broader than communication objectives, but must also specify outcomes.

Promotional mix: The combination of marketing techniques chosen in pursuit of a particular promotional goal.

Promotion: Any means of informing the marketplace that the organization has developed a response to meet its needs and includes the mechanisms available for facilitating the hoped-for exchange.

Provider: Generic term for a health professional or organization that provides direct patient care or related support services.

PSA: A public service announcement; an advertisement that a mass media outlet (e.g., magazine, newspaper, radio station, television station, Web site, outdoor venue) prints or broadcasts without charging the sponsoring organization.

Psychographics: The lifestyle characteristics of a population that include such factors as attitudes, consumer purchase patterns, and leisure activities, that can be used for determining communication styles.

Public relations: A form of communication management that seeks to make use of publicity and other non-paid forms of promotion and information to influence feelings, opinions or beliefs about the organization and its offerings.

Qualitative research: Subjective research that involves obtaining reactions and impressions from small numbers of people by engaging them in discussions. Qualitative research is useful for exploring reactions and uncovering additional ideas, issues, or concerns.

Quantitative research: Research designed to gather objective information by asking a large number of people identical (and predominantly closed-ended) questions. Quantitative research is useful for measuring the extent to which knowledge, attitudes, or behaviors are prevalent in an intended audience.

Reach: The number of people or households exposed to a specific media message during a specific period of time.

Readability testing: Use of a formula to predict the approximate reading level (usually expressed in grades) a person must have achieved in order to understand written material.

Recall: In pretesting, a measure that describes the extent to which respondents remember seeing or hearing a message that was shown in a competitive media environment—usually centers on recall of the main idea, not the verbatim message.

Relationship management: An approach to marketing that focuses on the maintenance of a long-term relationship between the buyer and seller and not on a one-time sale.

Relationship marketing: An approach to marketing that emphasizes the establishment and nurturing of long-term relationships rather than a one-time sale.

Reliability: Refers to communication content that is credible in terms of its source and its currency.

Repetition: Delivery of and access to content continued or repeated over time, both to reinforce the impact with a given audience and to reach new generations.

Return on investment (ROI): The benefits—however measured—returned to an organization as a result of its investment in a communication initiative.

Risk communication: Engaging communities in discussions about environmental and other health risks and about approaches to deal with them. Risk communication also includes individual counseling about genetic risks and consequent choices.

Sales: An approach to business that emphasizes the transactional aspects of the buyer-seller relationship rather than the more information-oriented approach associated with marketing.

Sales promotion: An activity or material that acts as a direct inducement by offering added value to the product or incentives for resellers, salespersons or consumers.

Sample survey: A data collection method that involves the administration of a survey form or questionnaire to a segment of a target population that has been systematically selected.

Secondary research: The analysis of data originally collected for some other purpose than its use for communication research.

Service area: The actual or desired area (usually defined in terms of geography) from which an organization draws or intends to draw its customers; often used interchangeably with "market area" but more commonly used by not-for-profit organizations.

Segment: A component of a population or market defined based on some characteristic relevant for communication.

Segmentation: Subdividing an overall population into homogeneous subsets in order to better describe and understand a group, predict behavior, and tailor messages and programs to match specific interests, needs, or other group characteristics.

Service: An intangible product that involves an activity or process (or sets thereof) carried out by a service provider that meets the needs of the consumer.

Setting: Times, places, and states of mind during which an intended audience is attentive and open to a message.

Social cognitive theory: A theory of human behavior that stresses the dynamic interrelationships among people, their behavior, and their environment.

Social marketing: The application and adaptation of commercial marketing concepts to the planning, development, implementation, and evaluation of programs that are designed to bring about behavior change to improve the welfare of individuals or communities.

Stages-of-change model: A theoretical framework that explains behavior change as a process rather than as an event. The model identifies individuals at various stages of readiness to attempt, to make, and to sustain a behavior change.

Strategic plan: A comprehensive plan for the organization that lays out its strategic direction.

Strategy: The generalized approach that is to be taken in meeting the challenges to communication.

Survey research: A category of data collection techniques that involves the use of a questionnaire or survey instrument administered in any one of a number of methods.

SWOT analysis: An approach to assessing an organization that examines its strengths and weaknesses as well as the opportunities and threats that confront it.

Synthetic data:	Data generated in the form of estimates, projections and forecasts that represent calculated figures as opposed to actual data.
Tailored communication:	Messages crafted for and delivered to each individual based on individual needs, interests, and circumstances.
Tailoring:	The process of creating messages and materials to reach one specific person based on characteristics unique to that person.
Target audience:	*See* intended audience.
Target marketing:	Marketing initiatives that focus on a market segment to which an organization desires to offer goods/services.
Targeting:	Creating messages and materials intended to reach a specific segment of a population, usually based on one or more demographic or other characteristics shared by its members.
Telemarketing:	The use of telephones for selling by means of either outbound or inbound calls.
Telemedicine:	The use of electronic information and communication technologies to provide clinical care across distance.
Telephone interview:	A data collection technique that involves the administration of a survey instrument by an interviewer to a respondent via the telephone.
Third-party payer:	A party other than the provider (seller) and patient (buyer) who pays for the cost of goods and/or services, usually an insurance company or government-sponsored health plan; also referred to as third-party payor.
Timeliness:	Content that is provided or available when the audience is most receptive to, or in need of, the specific information.

Trade show: The convening of interested parties related to a particular product or industry at which vendors can present their products.

Underserved: Individuals or groups who lack access to health services or information relative to the national average.

Understandability: Reading or language level and format (including multimedia) appropriate for a specific audience.

Up-selling: A process that involves convincing a buyer to choose a more extensive (and inevitably higher priced) product over the less complex choice.

Value: Anything that a society considers important, usually an intangible such as youth, economic success, education, or freedom.

Want: An expressed desire for a health service based on felt need on the part of the consumer rather than a medically identified need; a health service want may or may not correlate with a health service need.

Website: A location on the World Wide Web containing documents or files. Each site is owned and managed by an individual, company, or organization.

Index